£28·00

3 8027 00373990

Library: 4
Class: SLC 257A SAC
Acc: 13093
Date: 24/12/92

WITHDRAWN

GCNM LIBRARY	
Division East	No. 614.5992 AC S10
Dynix No. 50972	No. 324076
DATE 24/10/95	D PRICE £28-00

Eastern College of Nursing Library

Eastern College of Nursing Library
110 St James Road
GLASGOW G4 0PS

Tel: 041 552 1562 Ext. 2148/9

CLINICAL OBSTETRICS: A PUBLIC HEALTH PERSPECTIVE

Edited by

Benjamin P. Sachs, MB.BS, DPH(C)
and
David Acker, MD

LIBRARY
WESTERN COLLEGE
OF NURSING & MIDWIFERY
GARTNAVEL COMPLEX
1053 GREAT WESTERN ROAD
GLASGOW G12

PSG PUBLISHING COMPANY, INC.
LITTLETON, MASSACHUSETTS

Library of Congress Cataloging in Publication Data

Main entry under title:

Clinical obstetrics.

Includes index.
1. Obstetrics—Statistical methods—Addresses, essays, lectures. 2. Epidemiology—Addresses, essays, lectures. 3. Public health—Statistical methods—Addresses, essays, lectures.
I. Sachs, Benjamin P. II. Acker, David. [DNLM: 1. Epidemiologic Methods. 2. Obstetrics. WQ 100 C6413]
RG530.C57 1985 614.5′992 85-19079
ISBN 0-88416-513-2

Published by:
PSG PUBLISHING COMPANY, INC.
545 Great Road
Littleton, Massachusetts 01460

G. R. I.
...GE OF NURSING
LIBRARY
ACC. No. 23886
CLASS No. 25A
DATE M9 91
PRICE

Copyright © 1986 by PSG Publishing Company, Inc.

All rights reserved. No part of this publication may be reproduced or transmitted in any form or by any means, electronic or mechanical, including photocopy, recording, or any information storage or retrieval system, without permission in writing from the publisher.

Printed in the United States of America

International Standard Book Number: 0-88416-513-2

Library of Congress Catalog Card Number: 85-19079

Last digit is print number: 987654321

This book is affectionately dedicated to our wives, Vickie G. Sachs and Eva Skolnik-Acker. They know why.

CONTRIBUTORS

DAVID ACKER, MD
Assistant Professor
Obstetrics and Gynecology
Harvard Medical School
Associate Chief
Department of Obstetrics and Gynecology
Beth Israel Hospital
Boston

SUSAN BASSETT, MD
Instructor
Obstetrics and Gynecology
Harvard Medical School
Co-Director of Ambulatory Care
Department of Obstetrics and Gynecology
Beth Israel Hospital
Boston

LETITIA K. DAVIS, ScD, EdM
Senior Epidemiologist
Massachusetts Department of Public Health
Division of Health Statistics and Research
Research Fellow
Harvard University
Boston

ANDREW M. FRIEDE, MD, MPH
EIS Officer
Center for Health Promotion and Education
Division of Reproductive Health
Centers for Disease Control
Atlanta

TIMOTHY HEEREN, PhD
Assistant Professor
Epidemiology and Biostatistics
Boston University School of Public Health
Boston

L.B. HOLMES, MD
Associate Professor
Pediatrics
Harvard Medical School
Chief
Embryology Unit and Teratology Unit
Massachusetts General Hospital
Boston

JANINE M. JASON, MD
Chief
Epidemiology Studies
Division of Host Factors
Center for Infectious Diseases
Centers for Disease Control
Atlanta

JOHN FIGGIS JEWETT, MD
Professor of Clinical Obstetrics and Gynecology, Emeritus
Harvard Medical School
Former Chairman
Committee on Maternal Welfare, Massachusetts Medical Society
Former Director of Continuing Education
Brigham and Women's Hospital
Boston

HENRY KLAPHOLZ, MD
Assistant Professor
Obstetrics and Gynecology
Harvard Medical School
Co-Director
Divison of Maternal-Fetal Medicine
Beth Israel Hospital
Boston

GENE A. MCGRADY, MD
EIS Officer
Division of Host Factors
Center for Infectious Diseases
Centers for Disease Control
Atlanta

BARBARA R. POBER, MD
Fellow
Children's Service
Massachusetts General Hospital
Boston

ROGER W. ROCHAT, MD
Professor of Epidemiology
Emory University
Atlanta

SHARON L. ROSEN, PhD
Director
Division of Health Statistics and Research
Massachusetts Department of Public Health
Boston

MICHAEL ROSENBERG, MD, MPH
Director
Reproductive Epidemiology Division
Family Health International
Research Triangle Park, NC

BENJAMIN P. SACHS, MB.BS, DPH(C)
Assistant Professor
Obstetrics and Gynecology
Harvard Medical School and Harvard School of Public Health
Director
Division of Maternal-Fetal Medicine
Beth Israel Hospital
Boston

PHILLIP G. STUBBLEFIELD, MD
Associate Professor
Obstetrics and Gynecology
Harvard Medical School
Chairman
Department of Obstetrics and Gynecology
Mount Auburn Hospital
Cambridge

ISABELLE VALADIAN, MD
Professor
Maternal and Child Health
Harvard School of Public Health
Chairman
Department of Maternal and Child Health
Harvard School of Public Health
Boston

CONTENTS

FOREWORD **ix**

1 MATERNAL AND PERINATAL MORTALITY: AN EPIDEMIOLOGIC PERSPECTIVE **1**

Andrew M. Friede, MD, MPH, and Roger W. Rochat, MD

2 MATERNAL MORTALITY **35**

John Figgis Jewett, MD, and Benjamin P. Sachs, MB.BS, DPH(C)

3 EPIDEMIOLOGY OF PRETERM BIRTH **65**

Phillip G. Stubblefield, MD

4 ELECTRONIC FETAL MONITORING **93**

Henry Klapholz, MD, and Susan Bassett, MD

5 CESAREAN SECTION **119**

Letitia K. Davis, ScD, EdM, and Sharon L. Rosen, PhD

6 REPRODUCTIVE OUTCOME OF THE OLDER GRAVIDA **145**

David Acker, MD, and Benjamin P. Sachs, MB.BS, DPH(C)

7 CONGENITAL MALFORMATIONS: EPIDEMIOLOGY, DETECTION, AND PREVENTION **167**

Barbara R. Pober, MD, and L.B. Holmes, MD

8 REPRODUCTION AND THE WORKING ENVIRONMENT **205**

Michael Rosenberg, MD, MPH

9 AN HISTORICAL PERSPECTIVE ON CONTROVERSIES SURROUNDING THE INTERNATIONAL CODE OF MARKETING OF BREAST-MILK SUBSTITUTES **233**

Janine M. Jason, MD, and Gene A. McGrady, MD

10 GROWTH AND DEVELOPMENT OF GIRLS **255**

Isabelle Valadian, MD

11 INTRODUCTORY STATISTICS FOR OBSTETRICIANS **273**

Timothy Heeren, PhD

INDEX **299**

LIBRARY
WESTERN COLLEGE
OF NURSING & MIDWIFERY
GARTNAVEL COMPLEX
1053 GREAT WESTERN ROAD
GLASGOW G12

FOREWORD

Obstetrics as a discipline stands at the confluence of a number of fields of study, each of which contributes to the fuller understanding of the benefits and risks of its practices. None has had a more pervasive ameliorating impact than epidemiology. Perhaps in no other medical specialty have epidemiological techniques been applied so often and with such favorable results. Yet the principles of epidemiology tend to be about as foreign to obstetricians as the nuances of obstetrical problems are to epidemiologists.

Here then is an important volume to bridge the chasm. It not only offers substantive information on a number of extremely relevant and timely topics of mutual interest, but it delves in some depth into the shortcomings of available information and how to resolve pressing issues by more appropriate data collection and analytical methods.

The editors have brought their multidisciplinary backgrounds to bear to ensure against parochialism and redundancy and, at the same time, to guarantee relative homogeneity of approach throughout to make a cohesive whole. To say their task was not easy is clearly an understatement. Moreover, they have succeeded admirably. They have gathered recognized experts with diverse interests to work together in these pages toward the common goal of providing enlightenment in an area hitherto often illuminated only poorly and intermittently at best.

Although many of the issues addressed are controversial and some even highly inflammatory, the contributing authors have avoided hyperbole and the temptation to become shrill and vitriolic. Instead, they offer carefully framed presentations of facts and their limitations, of experimental design and data analysis and their deficiencies, and of problems associated with interpretations and conclusions stemming from those analyses. Their well-tempered and appropriately critical discussions are especially worthy of note. These reviews cross disciplinary lines and should, therefore, be read and digested by both obstetrical and public health specialists for whom they will prove valuable.

Given that public health policy pertaining to these issues will undoubtedly be made in the foreseeable future, it is essential for all to be made aware of the limitations of currently available data and the real need for further study. This applies especially to those in position to be policymakers or to influence them, as well as to practitioners of obstetrics and administrators and others who will be called upon to carry out the mandates of public health policy.

The messages of this book also apply across international borders both for developing and industrialized nations. While interested parties in industrialized countries debate the cost-effectiveness of high-technology developments in medical practice, they can learn much from the advances being made in emerging nations by the impressive gains resulting from small, but significant, changes in care practices. Those in developing countries can benefit in turn from data showing substantive value from (or more important, lack of advantage to) some of the new technological advances. In the overview, it is clear that there is need for this book. It deserves to be widely read.

Emanuel A. Friedman, MD, ScD
Boston, 1985

ACKNOWLEDGMENT

It is with a deep appreciation that we acknowledge Martha's patience and hard work. Without her this project would not have been possible.

CHAPTER 1

MATERNAL AND PERINATAL MORTALITY: AN EPIDEMIOLOGIC PERSPECTIVE

Andrew M. Friede, MD, MPH
Roger W. Rochat, MD

INTRODUCTION

The Surgeon General's *Objectives for the Nation* states that: "Assuring all infants a healthy start in life and enhancing the health of their mothers are among the highest priorities in preventing disease and promoting health."[1] The high priority given to maternal and infant health, plus steady declines from 1965 to 1978 in the US maternal mortality rate (Figure 1-1) and the perinatal mortality rates (Figure 1-2) led to the establishment of the following objectives. The objective for the maternal mortality rate (MMR), defined as the number of deaths due to complications of pregnancy, childbirth, and the puerperium per 100,000 live births, was: "By 1990, the maternal mortality rate should not exceed 5 per 100,000 live births for any county or any ethnic group (eg, black, Hispanic, American Indian). The objective for the perinatal mortality rate (PMR), defined as the number of late fetal deaths (at 28 weeks gestation or more) plus neonatal deaths at under 7 days of age, per 1000 live births plus late fetal deaths, was: "By 1990, the perinatal mortality rate should be reduced to no more than 5.5 per 1000."

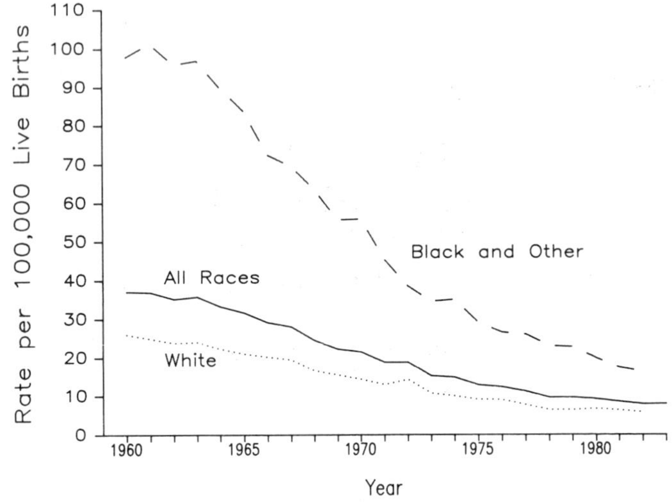

Figure 1-1 Maternal mortality rate by race: United States, 1960–1983. Source: NCHS (1984)[18] and NCHS, Division of Vital Statistics (personal communication).

If the 1990 objectives are to be met, obstetricians and public health planners will need to identify those groups at elevated risk of maternal and perinatal deaths and to develop prevention strategies targeted at the conditions that cause these deaths. This will require an improved scientific understanding of the epidemiology of these tightly linked subjects. This chapter summarizes the current epidemiology of maternal mortality and perinatal mortality in the United States. The first half reviews some definitions of maternal mortality, current data sources, and the epidemiology of the three principal components of maternal mortality: induced abortion, ectopic pregnancy, and childbearing. The second half reviews the definitions relevant to perinatal mortality, current data sources, and its epidemiology.

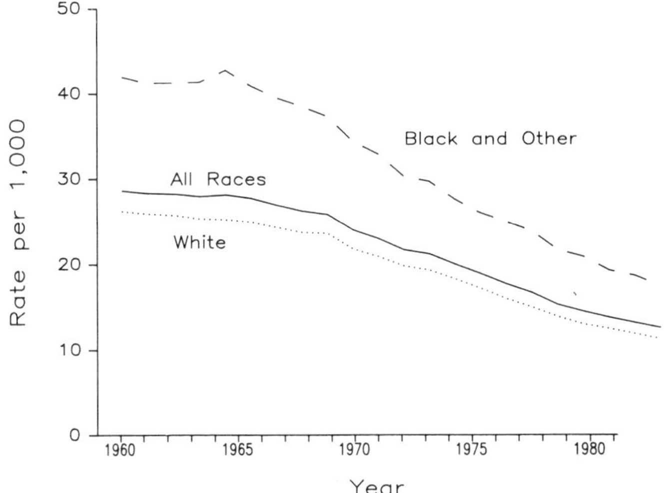

Figure 1-2 Perinatal mortality rate by race: United States, 1960–1981. The rate is calculated as the number of late fetal deaths (28 weeks or more gestation) plus early neonatal deaths (deaths at 0–6 days of age) per 1000 live births plus late fetal deaths. Source: NCHS (1984),[18] and NCHS, Division of Vital Statistics.

MATERNAL MORTALITY

Definitions

Some widely used definitions pertaining to maternal mortality are summarized in Table 1-1. Uniform definitions should provide the obstetrician and health planner with tools to identify groups at special risk, and facilitate comparisons between such groups, eg, mothers with different medical conditions, of different races, with different socioeconomic status, or living in different areas.

From this point of view, the current definitions have four important shortcomings. First, the definitions combine all maternal deaths, without regard to cause. This blurs the

Table 1-1
Definitions for Maternal Mortality

Maternal Death

Maternal death is the death of any woman, from any cause, while pregnant or within 42 days of termination of pregnancy, irrespective of the duration and the site of pregnancy.

Direct maternal death: An obstetric death resulting from obstetric complications of the pregnancy state, labor, or puerperium and from interventions, omissions, incorrect treatment, or chain of events resulting from any of these complications.

Indirect maternal death: An obstetric death resulting from previously existing disease, or disease that developed during pregnancy, labor, or the puerperium. It is not directly due to obstetric causes, but it is aggravated by the physiologic effects of pregnancy.

Nonmaternal death: An obstetric death resulting from accidental or incidental causes not related to the pregnancy or its management.

Maternal mortality rate (MMR)

ACOG*; AMA†: Number of maternal deaths (direct, indirect, or nonmaternal) per 100,000 terminated pregnancies.

NCHS‡; WHO§: Number of maternal deaths (direct and indirect) per 100,000 live births.

*American College of Obstetrics & Gynecology.[52]
†American Medical Association.[56]
‡National Center for Health Statistics.[34]
§World Health Organization.[53]

distinction between three very different outcomes of pregnancy: induced abortion, ectopic pregnancy, and childbearing. (Trophoblastic disease is a fourth, but different, sort of outcome. Its epidemiology has been recently reviewed, and will not be further considered here.[2]) Second, the definition of "maternal death" is time-limited to those occurring during a pregnancy, or within 42 days of its termination. This restriction probably has its origin in standard obstetrical care and the timing of the final postpartum visit. However, its use may cause many deaths related to pregnancy to be overlooked. For instance, in Georgia during 1974–1975, 22 of 76 (29%) deaths related to pregnancy that were identified by linked infant–maternal death records occurred after this 42-day cutoff.[3]

Third, the distinction between direct and indirect maternal deaths is not helpful for understanding the epidemiology of pregnancy. Although this categorization was designed to help estimate the degree to which a death was predictable or preventable, its capacity to do so has not been evaluated. Furthermore, these definitions are difficult to apply in a consistent fashion. For example, pyelonephritis can be classified as a direct, indirect, or nonmaternal death; pulmonary thromboembolism has been called "direct" in one report, but "indirect" in others.[4] Fourth, it may be extremely difficult to decide whether a death associated with pregnancy is maternal or nonmaternal, in part because of the poorly defined epidemiology of some causes of death. For example, it is unknown if pregnancy increases the risk of death due to homicide, suicide, or unintentional injury. Until more is known about the relationship of pregnancy to violence and injury, the classification of a death as "maternal" or "nonmaternal" will remain unreliable.

The choice of denominator for the calculation of the mortality rate deserves comment. Because the numerator in the American College of Obstetricians and Gynecologists and American Medical Association definition includes pregnancies with abortive outcomes, the use of terminated pregnancies as a denominator is appropriate. By contrast, the National Center for Health Statistics and World Health Organization currently use live births as the denominator, which excludes many of thc outcomes reflected in the numerator (abortions and ectopic pregnancies). This second method tends to make the apparent rate higher than the true rate.

With slight modification, the ACOG definitions could better serve the study of risk factors for maternal mortality. First, although ideally the definition of maternal death should be extended to include deaths up to one year after the termination of pregnancy, a 90-day cutoff would capture almost 95% of maternal deaths and would be easier to implement.[5] Second, the unreliable direct/indirect and maternal/nonmaternal classification methods should be replaced with detailed case inquires and epidemiologic investigations that would determine which deaths are preventable with current medical knowledge and whether they can be attributed to pregnancy.

Third, we need to develop several different kinds of maternal mortality rates to meet our current diverse needs. For areas with poor data about the number of pregnancies, the current definitions will approximate the risk of childbearing, and will be especially useful for comparisons with developing countries. Where better data are available, a "pregnancy mortality rate," defined as the number of deaths to pregnant women per 100,000 pregnancies, would be useful for evaluating the risk of pregnancy relative to the risk of contraception (ie, the risk of avoiding pregnancy). For prospective epidemiological studies, a "childbearing mortality rate," defined as the number of deaths to women who know they are pregnant, and who continue the pregnancy, per 100,000 births (fetal deaths plus live births), would be useful for comparing the value of alternative prenatal care strategies, or for comparison to the risk of elective abortion.[6] Different rates could be developed to serve specific purposes, just as death-to-case rates have been developed for deaths due to abortions and ectopic pregnancies.[6,7] In sum, we need to include in both numerator and denominator pregnancies and outcomes that match and that are of interest. However, these new measures will only be as accurate as their components. Accurate numerators require a complete count of pregnancy-associated deaths. We now review the sources of these data.

Data Sources

Vital records Historically, population-based studies of maternal mortality have depended on vital statistics data. These data are abstracted from death certificates, collated at the state level, and summarized and analyzed by individual states, and by NCHS. Unfortunately, a large number of maternal deaths are not detected by the vital records system; estimates of underreporting range from 17 to 73% (Table 1-2).

Underreporting is due to three principal factors. First, some maternal deaths are never diagnosed as such. This may be due in part to the fact that autopsies are not routine. The physician who attended a woman at death may not be aware that she was recently pregnant, and there is no systematic way for this information to be made available.

Second, even maternal deaths diagnosed as such may not be captured by the vital records system. The Centers for Disease Control (CDC) abortion surveillance system captures 59% more abortion-related deaths than do vital records alone.[8] No such system exists for childbearing deaths. Hence, both the quality and quantity of data vary widely by mortality category. Only five states have a space on the death certificate to indicate a recent pregnancy and, to our knowledge, no states routinely link birth records to the death records of women of childbearing age to detect maternal deaths. For Georgia during 1975–1976, a special linkage was responsible for capturing eight of 30 (27%) maternal deaths that occurred within 42 days of the termination of pregnancy (Table 1-2). When the definition of maternal death was extended to include deaths that occurred within one year of delivery, 12 of 36 (33%) maternal deaths were discovered exclusively by record linkage.[3] As the duration of time from delivery to death increased, the record linkage method became more important (Figure 1-3).

Third, the use of vital records as the source of epidemiologic data is inevitably associated with misclassifica-

Table 1-2
Number of Maternal Deaths by Method of Reporting

Years	Region	Source of new data	Vital records alone	Vital records plus new source	Percent under-reported	Reference
1974–1975	New Jersey	Active surveillance	30	52	42	Ziskin et al, 1979[55]
1975–1976	Georgia	Record linkage	22	30	27	Rubin et al, 1981[3]*
1978–1979	Puerto Rico	Death certificate review	4	15	73	Speckhard, 1981[54]
1974–1978	United States	State health department reports; certificate reviews	1949	2349	17	Smith et al, 1984[13]

*For the table, only maternal deaths within 42 days are included.

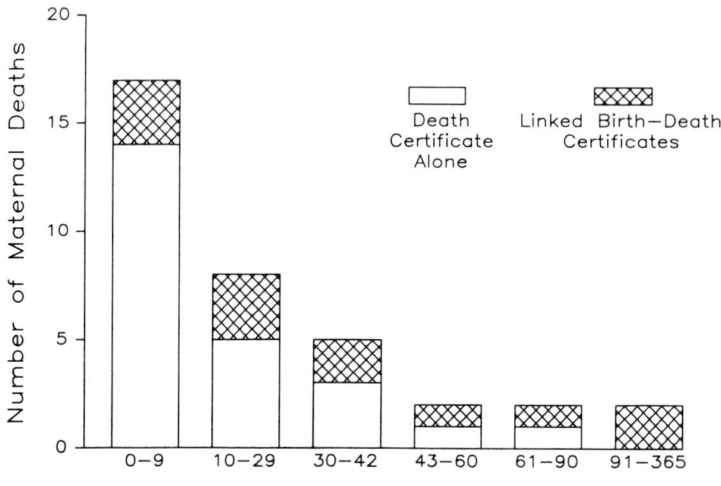

Figure 1-3 Number of maternal deaths by method of detection ($N = 36$): Georgia, 1975–1977. Source: Modified from data in Rubin et al (1981).[3]

tion.[9] However, even if the vital records system functioned perfectly, as currently designed, it cannot furnish the detail that is required to fully understand the epidemiology of maternal deaths. Vital statistics data are not timely, nor do they provide the detail required for a more complete understanding of the causal sequence of maternal mortality. For example, birth and death certificates often lack information on complications of pregnancy and associated therapies, smoking, alcohol and drug abuse, complications at delivery, and the participation of alternative health care providers. Similarly, unless they are linked to other data, they cannot provide data on long-term morbidity, nor on the consequences of maternal mortality and morbidity for the subsequent health of the child.

However, with some modifications, vital records could serve as a better source of epidemiologic data. First and foremost, linking birth records to maternal and infant death records, and to hospital discharge data, could provide valuable data on maternal outcomes. Second, to identify unreported maternal deaths, death certificates of all women of reproductive age should be reviewed by state health departments. Finally, continuing education of physicians should emphasize the importance of noting maternity-related causes of death on death certificates.

Surveillance To improve the availability of data on two components of maternal mortality—deaths due to abortion and deaths due to ectopic pregnancy—CDC has instituted national surveillance. There is no equivalent Federal surveillance of childbearing deaths. Hence, the quality and quantity of data vary widely by mortality category.

Abortion reporting The legalization of elective abortion made it urgent to improve our scientific understanding of abortion-related morbidity and mortality. This required better information. In 1969, CDC began a highly intensive national surveillance system for abortion.[8,10] This system provides complete data on abortion mortality, plus the detailed demographic and medical characteristics required to give these data meaning. For the period 1972–1980, 37% of the confirmed abortion-related deaths were reported through these supplemental sources. In addition to using vital statistics from state health departments, the CDC system gathers reports of abortion-related deaths from medical and hospital associations, maternal mortality committees, the NCHS, the Commission on Professional and Hospital Activities, case histories published in professional journals, and private sources. After confirmation, the CDC staff interviews the attending physician and reviews the records. When necessary, CDC investigators interview other health-care providers, friends, and relatives to identify factors than may have contributed to the death. Such factors have included the lack of local services, a woman's inability to pay for them, and personal behaviors.

The CDC has used this unique and complete data set in two ways. First, much in the manner of maternal mortality committee reports, the publication of careful case studies has alerted obstetricians to unusual complications, and to possible deficiencies in local practice. Second, in the style of classical investigative epidemiology, the analysis of this case series has identified groups at special risk for abortion mortality, eg, those having late abortions, undergoing hysterectomy/hysterotomy, and those who have illegal abortions. Information from the national abortion surveillance system has been widely disseminated. This may account, in part, for changes in obstetrical practice, and for the very rapid decline in mortality due to elective abortion.

Ectopic pregnancy reporting In 1979, CDC began surveillance of ectopic pregnancies.[11,12] This surveillance was prompted by the more than doubling of the ectopic pregnancy rate (the number of ectopic pregnancies per 1000 reported pregnancies) in the preceding decade and by the lack of comprehensive national data to understand this trend. The methods used for ectopic pregnancy surveillance differ somewhat from those used for abortion surveillance. Numbers of ectopic pregnancies are derived from the National Hospital Discharge Survey, which samples medical records from a representative sample of US hospitals. Deaths from ectopic pregnancies are identified by state health departments from a review of death certificates. These deaths are reported to CDC, which then conducts a detailed review of each case. Some of the important findings yielded by this system are described in the next section of this chapter.

Childbearing mortality reporting There is no formal national surveillance system for this third component of maternal mortality, which includes 84% of all maternal deaths. To test whether collecting data at the national level would produce useful results, CDC recently reviewed the death certificates (obtained directly from each state) for all US maternal deaths for 1974–1978, and compared them to

NCHS data.[13] This study found a 17% underreporting of maternal deaths as data proceeds from the state to the national level (Table 1-2), which suggests that routine Federal vital statistics underreport childbearing mortality.

Epidemiology

Trends over time From 1950 to 1978, the MMR dropped from 83.2 to 9.6 maternal deaths per 100,000 live births.[14] This decline has been attributed to new medical knowledge and its wide application; the increased availability of contraception; and safe, legal, elective abortion.[15,16] However, since 1981, the MMR has remained relatively stable. There were an estimated 290 maternal deaths in 1983, leading to a provisional MMR of 8.0; this rate is not significantly different than the final 1981 rate of 8.5 or the final 1982 rate of 7.9.[17–19] Reasons for the current slower decline include the possibility that the current maternal cohort is at higher risk of death; alternately, there may be improvement in preventing death from the current leading causes, or a real improvement that has been masked by improved reporting.

Some insight into this leveling off may be gained from an investigation of historical trends in maternal deaths by category (Figure 1-4). From 1970 to 1980, the proportion of maternal deaths due to induced abortion decreased from 8% to 2%, and that due to ectopic pregnancy increased from 8% to 14%; the proportion due to childbearing has remained stable at 84%. From 1972 to 1981, the annual number of legal abortions increased from 587,000 to 1,301,000; during this same period, the death-to-case rate declined from 4.1 to 0.5 per 100,000 abortions.[10] From 1970 to 1980, the annual number of ectopic pregnancies increased from 4.5 to 10.5 per 1000 reported pregnancies, but the death-to-case ratio decreased from 350 to 90 deaths per 100,000 ectopic pregnancies.[12] With respect to childbearing, from 1970 to 1980, the number of live births decreased slightly from 3,731,000 to

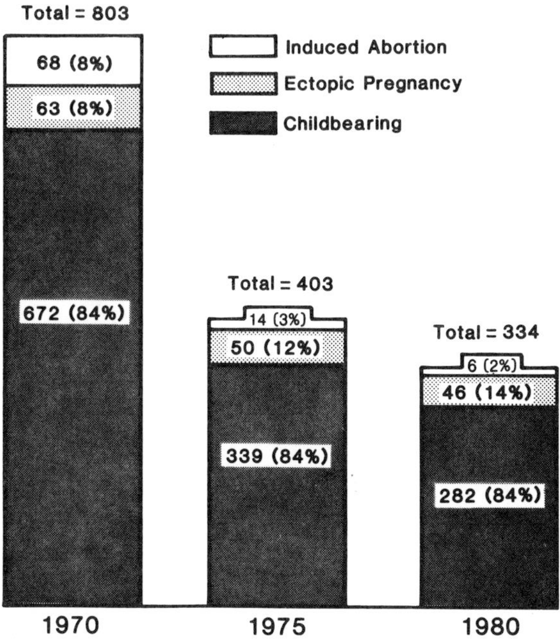

Figure 1-4 Maternal deaths by category: United States, 1970–1980. Source: NCHS (1974, 1977, 1984).[18,20,33]

3,629,000, with a nadir of 3,137,000 in 1973.[18] During this same period, the rate of maternal deaths due to childbearing declined from 18.0 to 7.8 per 100,000 live births.[17,20] In summary, the proportionate contribution of ectopic pregnancy is increasing and that due to elective abortion has declined rapidly; the absolute rate of childbearing deaths has declined, but not as a proportion of all maternal deaths.

Maternal characteristics In 1982, the overall MMR for whites was 5.8, compared with 18.2 for blacks; the relative risk was 3.1 (95% confidence limits = 2.5, 3.9).[21] Blacks have had consistently higher MMRs than whites, an effect that persists across all age groups (Figure 1-5).[4,16,22] Other risk

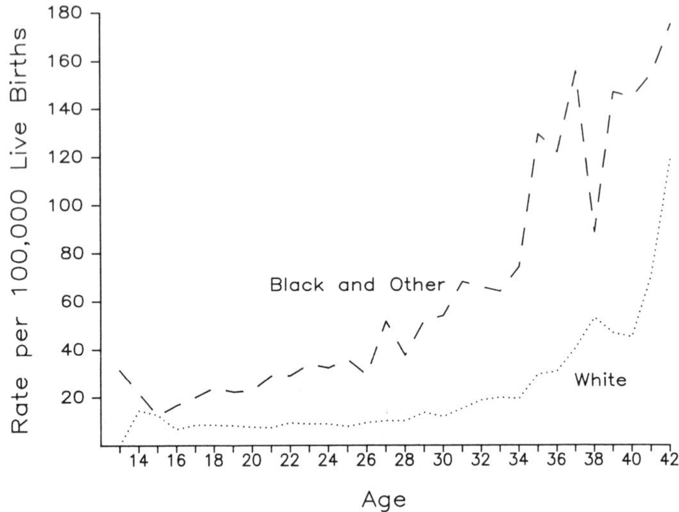

Figure 1-5 Maternal mortality rates by age and race: United States, 1974–1978. Source: CDC, unpublished data.

factors for an elevated MMR in the United States include extremes of age, and delivery in hospitals with very few or very many births per year.[16,23] These traditional findings have been confirmed by the CDC review of all 2475 US direct and indirect maternal death certificates for 1974–1978.[4] A recent finding from this research is that the traditional association of higher MMR with southern residency disappears when race is controlled (Table 1-3).

In contrast to the overall MMR, the death-to-case rate for abortion increases steadily with increasing age. Furthermore, blacks are at over twice the risk of whites.[7] For ectopic pregnancies, death-to-case rates do not vary much by age, ranging from 1.6 to 1.9 per 1000 ectopic pregnancies. The risk of death for blacks plus other minorities is 3.4 times the risk for whites.[24] The death-to-case rate is highest in the South and lowest in the West; as is true for maternal

Table 1-3
Maternal Deaths and Maternal Mortality Rates per 100,000 Live Births by Race and Region: United States, 1974–1978*

	Race					
	White		*Black and other*		*All*	
Region	Number	MMR	Number	MMR	Number	MMR
Northeast	233	8.8	195	39.9	436	13.9
Northcentral	411	10.9	249	43.1	661	15.2
South	431	10.8	546	38.6	977	18.0
West	300	10.9	101	24.9	401	12.7
Total	1375	10.5	1091	37.8	2475	15.4

*Source: CDC, unpublished data.

mortality in general, most of the geographic variation is attributable to geographic differences in racial distribution.[24]

Given that childbearing deaths account for 84% of maternal deaths, it is not surprising that childbearing deaths reflect the demographic features of overall maternal mortality. Women under 20 and over 29 are at higher risk; women over 34 are at the very highest risk. The risk of death for blacks plus other minorities is almost three times the risk for whites.[7]

Causes of death Historically, the important causes of maternal death have been hypertensive disease of pregnancy, hemorrhage, and infection. Low autopsy rates contribute to uncertainty as to the causes of death. Of reported maternal deaths in the United States during 1973–1975, 61% were autopsied. Women who were older, black, living in nonmetropolitan areas, living in the South, or whose deaths were attributed to toxemia or hemorrhage, were less likely to have had autopsies.[16]

Data from the CDC abortion surveillance system for 1979–1981 demonstrated that the most common causes of death for the 36 fatalities were: complications of anesthesia (33%), hemorrhage (19%), embolus (all types) (17%), and infection (14%). Data from the ectopic surveillance system for 1979–1980 demonstrated that the most common causes of deaths for the 86 ectopic pregnancy-related fatalities were: hemorrhage (85%), infection (5%), and anesthesia (2%).[25] Case investigation of ectopic pregnancy deaths during 1979–1980 found that of 48 deaths for which details of medical care were known, 33 (69%) might have been prevented if physicians had acted more appropriately; the other 15 (31%) might have been averted if the patient had sought care sooner.[25] For pregnancies not associated with an abortive outcome, there are detailed data available from the CDC for 1974–1978. For this study, the underlying cause of death was determined by the critical review of death certificates

Table 1-4
Causes of Maternal Deaths: United States, 1974–1978*

	Number	Percent
Pregnancies not associated with an abortive outcome		
Embolism	491	19.8
Hypertensive disease	421	16.9
Obstetric hemorrhage	331	13.4
Obstetric infection	196	7.9
Cerebrovascular accident	111	4.5
Anesthesia/analgesia complications	98	4.0
Other and unspecified causes of maternal death	419	16.9
Total	2067	83.4
Pregnancies with an abortive outcome		
Ectopic pregnancy	254	10.3
abortion	141	5.7
Gestational trophoblastic disease	16	0.6
Total	411	16.6
All causes	**2478**	**100.0**

*Source: Kaunitz[4].

by an obstetrician–gynecologist/epidemiologist.[4] Using this method, Kaunitz et al[4] found that embolism is now the leading cause of childbearing deaths, followed by the traditional triad (Table 1-4). The new prominence of embolism could be due to the use of this new classification method or to a relatively slower decline in embolic deaths, as compared to deaths from other causes. Amniotic fluid embolus, which accounted for 38% of the embolic deaths, is a diagnosis that is difficult to verify or refute at autopsy, and so is unlikely to lead to litigation. It has been suggested that this may tend to make it overreported.[4]

PERINATAL MORTALITY

Definitions

Some widely used definitions for perinatal and infant mortality are summarized in Table 1-5. Perinatal mortality began to receive increasing attention after 1955, when it became clear that much of this century's decline in infant mortality was due to infant deaths that occurred after the perinatal period.[26] There are two advantages to combining late fetal and early neonatal deaths into a single period of observation. First, it obviates the inevitable misclassifications that result from the difficulty inherent in deciding what is truly a live birth. Second, by removing a somewhat arbitrary distinction, it focuses attention on a period that is of joint interest to obstetricians and pediatricians; its wider use may encourage collaboration.[27]

However, from the point of view of facilitating comparisons between studies and countries of women whose pregnancies are at high risk of perinatal death, some of the current definitions of perinatal mortality may have shortcomings. First, the NCHS definitions do not offer guidance on the exclusion of fetal deaths that are likely to be under 28 weeks of gestation. For completeness, NCHS also published a PMR-II, which includes fetal deaths of 20 weeks gestation and all neonatal deaths, and a PMR-III, which includes these earlier fetal deaths, but early neonatal deaths only. Second, the perinatal mortality ratio excludes from the denominator many of the outcomes reflected in the numerator: late fetal deaths. The reported ratio will always give a higher value than the perinatal mortality rate (although in the strict statistical sense, this rate would be more accurately termed a *proportion*).

We have two recommendations. First, to facilitate comparisons, the United States should be able to prepare reports that use the standard WHO definitions. Unfortunately,

Table 1-5
Definitions for Perinatal Mortality

Live births
NCHS,* WHO† Live birth is complete expulsion or extraction from its mother of a product of conception, irrespective of the duration of the pregnancy, which, after such separation, breathes or shows any other evidence of life, such as beating of the heart, pulsation of the umbilical cord, or definite movement of voluntary muscles, whether or not the umbilical cord has been cut or the placenta is attached; each product of such a birth is considered live born.

Infant mortality rate
NCHS Number of infant deaths (deaths of infants under 1 year of age) per 1000 live births.

Neonatal mortality rate
NCHS Number of neonatal deaths (deaths of infants 0–27 days of age) per 1000 live births.

Postneonatal mortality rate
NCHS Number of postneonatal deaths (deaths of infants 28–365 days of age) per 1000 live births.

Perinatal mortality rate (PMR)
NCHS Number of late fetal deaths (fetal deaths of 28 weeks or more gestation) plus early neonatal deaths (deaths of infants 0–6 days of age) per 1000 live births plus fetal deaths.
WHO, National Number of fetuses and live births weighing at least 500 g [or when birth weight is unavailable, the corresponding gestational age (22 weeks) or body length (25 cm crown–heal)] dying before day 7 of life per 1000 such fetuses and infants.
WHO, International As above, but change minimum criteria for inclusion to 1000 g [or, where birth weight is unavailable, the corresponding gestational age (28 weeks) or body length (35 cm crown–heel)].

Perinatal mortality ratio
NCHS, WHO As above for their respective definitions, but exclude fetal deaths from the denominator.

*NCHS (1983).[34]
†WHO (1977);[53] UN (1982).[28]

because neither birth weight nor gestational age appears on the infant death certificate, the required data are currently unavailable; linked birth–death certificates may make this information available in the future (see next section). Second, the perinatal mortality ratio should be reserved for making comparisons with areas where information about the number of fetal deaths is highly unreliable; in fact, for international comparisons, the WHO reports the ratio.[28] An accurate estimate of the true perinatal mortality rate will require an improved count of late fetal deaths.

Data Sources

Each of the three components of the perinatal mortality rate (births, late fetal deaths, and early neonatal deaths) has a different degree of uncertainty associated with it. The registration of births in the United States is thought to be essentially complete; the very large number of births relative to deaths makes the PMR immune from the effect of the occasional unregistered birth. In contrast, the count of early neonatal deaths among high-risk groups is probably an underestimate. For example, deaths among infants with a Spanish surname in Texas[29] and of Asian origin in Washington State[30] have been thought to be undercounted. In North Carolina, a missing or erroneous gestational age was more common among births to young, unmarried, nonwhite mothers who had received less education and less prenatal care than controls.[31] In Georgia, the underregistration of neonatal deaths occurred disproportionately in rural areas, among unmarried mothers, and for black infants.[32] The pattern of these errors suggests that epidemiological analyses that rely on vital statistics may consistently underestimate the PMR of high-risk pregnancies.

The limitations of vital statistics data that apply to maternal mortality hold true for studying perinatal deaths. However, again, these data sources can be made more useful. Valuable information could be obtained from fetal death records linked to the death certificates of women of reproductive age and to hospital discharge data. In 1985, CDC will begin to analyze data from the National Infant Mortality Surveillance System, which will use tabular data prepared from linked birth and infant death certificates provided by states to derive the first national estimates of birth-weight-specific neonatal mortality available since 1960, and to describe the associated risk factors for neonatal death. The NCHS is currently evaluating proposals to link birth and infant death certificates at the national level. These new data sources should expand our understanding of the epidemiology of perinatal mortality.

Epidemiology

Trends over time From 1954 to 1964, the PMR remained fairly stable, declining from 30.2 to 28.4 perinatal deaths per 1000 live births, an average of only 0.6% per year. However, in 1965, the PMR began to drop steadily, by an average of 3.4% per year (Figure 1-2). In 1981, the last year for which data are available (no provisional data are reported for fetal deaths), there were 45,854 perinatal deaths, resulting in a PMR of 12.6, as compared to 13.2 in 1980.[18] The data limitations discussed above have undermined our ability to understand the cause of this decline.

However, insight into the national trends can be gained from two sources: (1) research on the decline in neonatal mortality, and (2) William's extensive studies of perinatal mortality in California. We can use these ancillary sources of information for the following reasons. The large degree of overlap between perinatal and neonatal deaths suggests that the explanation for the decline in neonatal mortality, in part, applies to the fall in perinatal mortality. In the United States during 1970–1980, over 55% of each year's perinatal deaths were neonatal deaths, and over 84% of neonatal deaths were early neonatal deaths (deaths during days 0–6 of life).[20,33,34] Because the California analyses evaluated the effect of many subgroups and risk factors one at a time, the results are likely to be relevant for similar groups in the United States as a whole. Over 80% of the decline in neonatal mortality in the United States has been attributed to lower birth-weight-specific infant mortality rates, with the remainder due to the moderate improvements in birth weight.[35–37] The improved survival of low-birth-weight infants is probably due to the introduction of neonatal intensive-care units and maternal transport.[37,38]

For the California analyses, the PMR included fetal deaths of 20 weeks' or more gestation and infant deaths during days 0–27 of life, and excluded any births weighing less than 501 g.[39a] The major findings were as follows. Approximately 70% of the decline in the PMR in California during 1960–1977 was attributable to improvement in the survival of neonates. Only 19% of the overall improvement in PMR was attributable to higher birth weights, but blacks did not benefit from higher birth weights at all. Moreover, increases in birth weight predicted an improvement in PMRs better than did proportionate increases in gestational age.[39b] Birth at hospitals that used electronic fetal monitoring in a high proportion of births and that had high cesarean section rates were also associated with declining PMRs.[39a,40] Medicaid recipients had lower PMRs than comparable nonrecipients; blacks and white, Spanish-surname Medicaid recipients had the most rapid decline in PMR.[41]

In summary, the decline of the US PMR during the 1970s was probably largely due to improved birth-weight-specific survival, which in turn has resulted from more sophisticated medical care and easier access to this care for minority groups. Further improvements will depend in part on developing a method to improve birth weights and prolong gestation.

Maternal factors Biological and socioeconomic effects place certain groups at risk for elevated PMRs. A recent analysis of Swedish data for 1976–1980 found that increasing maternal age and a history of prior fetal loss are independent predictors of higher rates of fetal and early neonatal mortality.[42] Compared to women aged 20–24, women aged 35–39 had double the risk of late fetal death. The implications for delayed childbearing are clear.

Low socioeconomic status is a strong predictor of neonatal mortality in the United States.[43] This effect has been found in many developed countries.[44] In 1981, the PMR for whites was 11.9, compared with 19.4 for blacks; the relative risk was 1.7 (95% confidence limits = 1.6, 1.8). Exactly how low socioeconomic status leads to perinatal death is unknown. It probably exerts its effect by lowering access to prenatal care[41] and by increasing the exposure to personal risk factors, eg, smoking, which is a strong predictor of perinatal mortality.[45] We urgently need research that will explain how socioeconomic status exerts its effect on perinatal survival.

Causes of death Because the sequence that leads to a perinatal death can be so complex, it may be difficult to accurately specify a single cause of death. Partly because of this, causes of fetal death (and hence, perinatal death) are not published by NCHS. However, causes of early neonatal death are available (Table 1-6), and causes of perinatal deaths are available from other countries and the United States Collaborative Perinatal Project (Table 1-7). Comparisons between these five studies must be made with caution; they covered different times and used varying methods. Some of the discrepancies between the Finnish and Japanese results can be attributed to differences in autopsy classification schemes. Much of what Nakamura et al[47] classified under asphyxia were actually complications of the cord and placenta. Bearing these caveats in mind, some general conclusions can be drawn.

First, conditions that lead to chronic anoxia continue to be important causes of perinatal death. Second, as deaths due to birth trauma become rare, congenital anomalies and respiratory distress syndrome are gaining new prominence.

Table 1-6
Early Neonatal Deaths (0–6 Days of Age) and Mortality Rates (per 100,000 Live Births) for Selected Causes of Death: United States, 1982*

	Number	Rate
All causes	23,706	640.0
Certain gastrointestinal diseases	10	0.3
Pneumonia and influenza	66	1.8
Congenital anomalies	5,415	146.2
Disorders relating to short gestation and unspecified low birth weight	3,542	95.6
Birth trauma	410	11.1
Intrauterine hypoxia and birth asphyxia	1,195	32.3
Respiratory distress syndrome	3,216	96.8
Other conditions originating in the perinatal period	9,020	243.5
Suddent infant death syndrome	79	2.1
All other causes	753	20.3

*Source: NCHS, Division of Vital Statistics (personal communication).

Finally, it is remarkable that even after autopsy, almost 10% of the causes of death remain unknown.

Other trends were noted in the individual studies. An evaluation of the trends in the causes of death in England and Wales for 1968–1978 attributed almost none of the decline in the PMR to a reduction in deaths due to maternal and fetal infections and medical conditions of the mother.[48] These investigators suggested that the introduction of intrapartum monitoring contributed to the decline in the role of anoxia. In Turku, Finland, from 1968 to 1982, PMRs for respiratory distress syndrome and asphyxia, cause unspecified, declined.[49] The Finnish investigations believe that these improvements are due to better services. Neither study was able to adequately address the possible contribution of changes in the important maternal factors described above.

SUMMARY AND RECOMMENDATIONS

We have argued that (1) the elaboration of the epidemiology of maternal and perinatal mortality requires timely, detailed data; (2) the vital statistics system is currently not well suited for this task; and (3) changes in the way vital statistics are reported, collated, and analyzed should make them more useful as sources of epidemiologic data. For abortion and ectopic pregnancy deaths, national surveillance has made it possible to gather detailed information about risk factors and current causes. However, we lack such a system for 84% of maternal deaths: those due to childbearing. Similarly, we have not had a national system for the surveillance for perinatal mortality.

For maternal mortality, the successful models of active national surveillance could be applied to childbearing mortality, with the institution of national maternal mortality surveillance. Case ascertainment could be improved by review of delivery logs, discharge summaries, the proceedings of hospital and state mortality committees, and medical examiners' reports. To augment these data, routine autopsies of women who die of maternal causes should be encouraged, and records of deaths among women of reproductive age should be linked to fetal death and birth and infant death records. These strategies would identify more cases of maternal deaths and also provide sufficient detail per case to understand what happened.

For perinatal mortality, the National Infant Mortality Surveillance System will be able to furnish national information about neonatal mortality, of which the perinatal period is such an important component. State perinatal audits could gather more detailed and more locally pertinent information. We need to better define which elements of prenatal care may contribute to lower perinatal mortality. Although surveillance systems that are centralized at the national level are feasible, they are not necessarily the most effective. Perhaps

Table 1-7
Perinatal Mortality Rates per 1000 and Proportion of Perinatal Deaths by Cause in Five Studies

	Vital records studies				Autopsy and record review studies					
	Norway 1967–1984 N = 1270 (approx.) (Bakketeig et al, 1984)*[26]		*England and Wales 1978 N = not specified (Edouard and Alberman, 1980)*[48]		*United States 1959–1966 N = 1435 (Naeye, 1977)*[46]		*Kurume, Japan† 1972–1979 N = 1000 (Nakamura et al, 1982)*[47]		*Turku, Finland† 1980–1982 N = 124 (Piekkala et al, 1985)*[49]	
Primary cause of death	PMR	Percent	PMR	Percent	PMR	Percent	PMR‡	Percent	PMR	Percent
Complications of cord and placenta	2.8	31	3.5	23	10.5	30	—		1.4	19
Birth trauma	2.8	31	0.9	6	0.6	2	—			
Prematurity	0.8	9	2.3	15	3.5	10	—	2		
Maternal complications during pregnancy	0.8	9	1.2	8			—	2	0.9	12
Congenital anomaly	0.7	8	3.5	23	2.9	8	—	20	1.6	21
Asphyxia, cause unspecified	0.7	8	1.5	10			—	14	0.2	3
Multiple pregnancy			0.7	4	0.3	1	—			
Maternal and fetal infection			0.3	2	6.2	17	—	28		
Erythroblastosis fetalis			0.2	1	1.5	4	—			
Fetal malnutrition					0.04	0.1	—		0.6	8

Respiratory distress syndrome							—	20	1.2	16
Other	0.5	5	1.5	9.8	2.5	7	—	7	0.9	12
Unknown					7.6	21	—	6	0.7	9
All	9.2	100	15.5	100	35.7	100	—	100	7.5	100

*Estimated from PMR applied to 138,182 births; all births were second births.
†Included late fetal deaths and neonatal deaths (0–27 days of age).
‡Not reported in this study.

a more productive method would be a cooperative effort that would include ACOG and its members, state health officials, and CDC. This model has worked well for the reporting of infectious diseases.

A similar system has been applied to maternal and perinatal mortality in Great Britain.[50] Since 1952, Great Britain's Department of Health and Social Security has made a "confidential inquiry" into every case of maternal death in England and Wales and periodic investigations of infant deaths. The area medical officer prepares a highly detailed, interpretive case report from records obtained from all health personnel who were involved. For each type of outcome, the current epidemiology is described in detail, and comparisons are made to previous years. Most importantly, investigators enumerate "avoidable factors" and make very specific recommendations. This rich and insightful analysis demonstrates how a detailed epidemiologic and interpretive inquiry into maternal and infant deaths can lead to practical recommendations. The United States should consider adopting similar methods.

CONCLUSION

Perhaps the central finding of epidemiologic research into maternal and perinatal mortality is that modern integrated care strategies are making a difference. Lest we forget this lesson, a recent tragedy will serve as further testimony.

The Faith Assembly religious group has been active in northeastern Indiana since 1973. Its tenets proscribe any medical care for its 2000 members. Reports of elevated fetal, neonatal, and maternal death rates prompted an investigation of maternal and perinatal mortality among this group for 1975–1982. Compared with other Indianans, Faith Assembly members had a relative risk of 92 for maternal mortality (95% confidence limits = 19, 280), and 2.7 for perinatal mortality 95% confidence limits = 1.6, 4.2).[51] This story should serve as a reminder that maternal and perinatal mortality are inextricably linked. Sustained progress in both areas will require improved access to modern obstetrical and neonatal care for minority groups and new efforts to better define which components of this care can prevent these deaths.

ACKNOWLEDGMENTS

We are grateful to Carol J. R. Hogue, PhD, Centers for Disease Control, and Ronald L. Williams, PhD, University of California, for reviewing the manuscript.

REFERENCES

1. US Public Health Service: *Objectives For the Nation.* Atlanta, Georgia, Public Health Service, 1980, p 17.
2. Grimes DA: Epidemiology of gestational trophoblastic disease. *Am J Obstet Gynecol* 1984;150:309–318.
3. Rubin G, McCarthy B, Shelton J, et al: The risk of childbearing re-evaluated. *Am J Public Health* 1981;71:712–716.
4. Kaunitz AM, Hughes JM, Grimes DA, et al: Causes of maternal mortality in the United States. *Obstet Gynecol* 1985;65: 605–612.
5. Rochat RW, Rubin GL, Selik R, et al: Changing the definition of maternal mortality: A new look at the postpartum interval (letter). *Lancet* 1981;(1):831.
6. Cates W Jr, Smith JC, Rochat RW, et al: Mortality from abortion and childbirth: Are the statistics biased? *JAMA* 1982;248: 192–196.
7. LeBolt SA, Grimes DA, Cates W Jr: Mortality from abortion and childbirth: Are the populations comparable? *JAMA* 1982;248: 188–192.
8. Centers for Disease Control: *Abortion Surveillance,* 1979–1980. Atlanta, Georgia, Public Health Service, 1983, pp 1–78.
9. Zemach R: What the vital statistics system can and cannot do. *Am J Public Health* 1984;74:756–758.
10. Centers for Disease Control: *Abortion Surveillance: Preliminary Analysis—United States, 1981.* Atlanta, 1984;MMWR33:373–375.
11. Centers for Disease Control: *Ectopic Pregnancy Surveillance,*

1970–1978. Atlanta, Georgia, Public Health Service, 1982, pp 1–19.
12. Centers for Disease Control: *Ectopic Pregnancies—United States, 1979–1980.* Atlanta, 1984;MMWR33:201–202.
13. Smith JC, Hughes JM, Pekow PS, et al: An assessment of the incidence of maternal mortality in the United States. *J Am Public Health* 1984;74:780–783.
14. National Center for Health Statistics: *Vital Statistics of the United States, 1979, vol II, Mortality, part A.* Washington, Public Health Service 1984, (DHSHS publications no (PHS) 84-1101), 1984.
15. Population Information Program: Healthier mothers and children through family planning. *Population Reports* 1984;12:J657–J696.
16. Rochat RW: Maternal and perinatal mortality statistics, in Silvio A (ed): *Obstetrical Practice.* St Louis, CV Mosby Co, 1980, pp 264–278.
17. National Center for Health Statistics: *Annual Summary of Births, Deaths, Marriages, and Divorces: United States, 1983.* Monthly Vital Statistics Report 32(13):1–24. Hyattsville, MD, Public Health Service, 1984 (DHHS publication no (PHS) 84-1120), 1984.
18. National Center for Health Statistics: *Advance Report of Final Natality Statistics.* Monthly Vital Statistics Report 32(9):Suppl. Hyattsville, MD, Public Health Service, 1983 (DHHS publication no (PHS) 84-1120), 1984.
19. National Center for Health Statistics: *Advance Report of Final Mortality Statistics, 1981.* Monthly Vital Statistics Report 33(3):Suppl. Washington, Public Health Service (DHHS publication no (PHS) 84-1120), 1984.
20. National Center for Health Statistics: *Final Mortality Statistics, 1970.* Monthly Vital Statistics Report 22(11):Suppl. Rockville, MD, Public Health Service (DHHS publication no. (HRA) 74-1120), 1974.
21. Rothman KJ, Boice JD: *Epidemiologic Analysis With a Programmable Calculator.* Boston, MA, Epidemiology Resources, Inc, 1982, p 16.
22. Schaffner Y, Federspiel CF, Fulton ML, et al: Maternal mortality in Michigan: An epidemiologic analysis, 1950–1971. *Am J Public Health* 1977;67:821–829.
23. Kaunitz AM, Grimes DA, Hughes JM, et al: Maternal deaths in the United States by size of hospital. *Obstet Gynecol* 1984;64:621–624.

24. Rubin GL, Peterson HB, Dorfman SF, et al: Ectopic pregnancy in the United States, 1970–78. *JAMA* 1983;249:725–729.
25. Dorfman SF, Grimes DA, Cates W Jr, et al: Ectopic pregnancy mortality, United States, 1979–80: Clinical aspects. *Obstet Gynecol* 1984;62:334–338.
26. Bakketeig LS, Hoffman HJ, Oakley ART: Perinatal mortality, in Bracken MB (ed): *Perinatal Epidemiology.* New York, Oxford University Press, 1984, pp 99–151.
27. Thompson AM, Barron SL: Perinatal Mortality, in Barron SL, Thompson AM (eds): *Obstetrical Epidemiology.* London, Academic Press, 1983, pp 347–398.
28. United Nations: *Demographic Yearbook, 1981.* New York, United Nations, 1982, p 39.
29. Powell-Griner E, Streck D: A closer examination of neonatal mortality rates among the Texas Spanish surname population. *Am J Public Health* 1982;72:993–999.
30. Frost F, Shy KK: Racial differences between linked birth and infant death records in Washington State. *Am J Public Health* 1980;70:974–976.
31. David RJ: The quality and completeness of birthweight and gestational age data in computerized birth files. *Am J Public Health* 1980;70:964–973.
32. McCarthy BJ, Terry J, Rochat RW, et al: The underregistration of neonatal deaths: Georgia 1974–1977. *Am J Public Health* 1980;70:977–982.
33. National Center for Health Statistics: *Final Mortality Statistics, 1975.* Monthly Vital Statistics Report 25(11):Suppl. Rockville, MD, Public Health Service (DHEW publication no (HRA) 77-1120), 1977.
34. National Center for Health Statistics: *Health, United States, 1983.* Washington, Public Health Service (DHHS publication no (PHS) 84-1232), 1983.
35. Lee K, Paneth N, Gardner LM, et al: Very low birth weight rate: Principal predictor of neonatal mortality in industrialized populations. *J Pediatr* 1980a;97:759–764.
36. Lee KS, Paneth N, Gardner LM, et al: Neonatal mortality: An analysis of the recent improvement in the United States. *Am J Public Health* 1980b;70:15–21.
37. McCormick MC: The contribution of low birth weight to infant mortality and childhood morbidity. *N Engl J Med* 1985;312:82–90.
38. David RJ, Siegel E: Decline in neonatal mortality, 1968 to 1977: Better babies or better care? *Pediatrics* 1983;71:531–540.

39a. Williams RL, Chen PM: Identifying the sources of the recent decline in perinatal mortality rates in California. *N Engl J Med* 1982;306:207–214.
39b. Williams RL, Creasy RK, Cunningham GC, et al: Fetal growth and perinatal viability in California. *Obstet Gynecol* 1982;59: 624–632.
40. Williams RL, Hawes WE: Cesarean section, fetal monitoring, and perinatal mortality in California. *Am J Public Health* 1979;69: 864–870.
41. Norris FD, Williams RL: Perinatal outcomes among Medicaid recipients in California. *Am J Public Health* 1984;74:1112–1117.
42. Forman MR, Merik O, Berendes HW: Delayed childbearing in Sweden. *JAMA* 1984;252:3135–3139.
43. Paneth N, Wallenstein S, Kiely L, et al: Social class indicators and mortality in low birth weight infants. *Am J Epidemiol* 1982;116:364–375.
44. World Health Organization: *Social and Biological Effect on Perinatal Mortality.* Budapest, Hungary, World Health Organization, 1978.
45. Meyer MB, Jonas BS, Tonascia JA: Perinatal events associated with maternal smoking during pregnancy. *Am J Epidemiol* 1976;103:464–476.
46. Naeye PL: Causes of perinatal mortality in the United States collaborative perinatal project. *JAMA* 1977;238:228–229.
47. Nakamura Y, Hosokawa Y, Yano H, et al: Primary causes of perinatal death: An autopsy study of 1,000 cases in Japanese infants. *Hum Pathol* 1982;13:4–62.
48. Edouard L, Alberman E: National trends in the certified causes of perinatal mortality. *Br J Obstet Gynecol* 1980;87:833–838.
49. Piekkala P, Erkkola R, Kero P, et al: Declining perinatal mortality in a region of Finland, 1968–1982. *Am J Public Health* 1985;75:156–160.
50. Tomlinson J, Turnbull A, Rudson G, et al: Report on confidential enquiries into maternal deaths in England and Wales 1973–1975. Report on health and social subjects. *HMSO* 1979;14:1–166.
51. Kaunitz AM, Spence C, Danielson TS, et al: Perinatal and maternal mortality in a religious group avoiding obstetric care. *Am J Obstet Gynecol* 1984;150:826–831.
52. American College of Obstetricians and Gynecologists: *Standards for Obstetric and Gynecologic Services.* Chicago, American College of Obstetrics and Gynecology, 1974, p 75.

53. World Health Organization: *Manual of the International Statistical Classification of Diseases, Injuries, and Causes of Death.* Geneva, World Health Organization, 1977, pp 763–766.
54. Speckhard ME: *Maternal Mortality Surveillance in Puerto Rico.* Presented at the 30th annual Epidemic Intelligence Service Conference, Centers for Disease Control, Atlanta, April 26, 1981.
55. Ziskin LZ, Gregory M, Kreitzer M: Improved surveillance of maternal deaths. *Int J Obstet Gynecol* 1979;16:281–286.
56. American Medical Association: *Action Guide for Maternal and Child Care Committees.* Chicago, American Medical Association, 1974, p 23.

CHAPTER 2

MATERNAL MORTALITY

John Figgis Jewett, MD
Benjamin P. Sachs, MB.BS, DPH(C)

INTRODUCTION

Death in childbirth has long troubled mankind. For millennia sudden unforeseen death of the young was an expected daily event and yet even then the sacrifice of one life to yield another was emotionally unacceptable. As early as 1470 in Sir Thomas Malory's *Morte D'Arthur*, a father's soliloquy records the poignancy of this tragedy: "Ah my little son thou hast murdered thy mother! . . . When he is christened let call him Tristam, that is as much to say as a sorrowful birth." Furthermore, beyond private suffering, the threat of maternal mortality to the public good was also recognized, for about the same time, Leonardo da Vinci recorded in his prophecies that "Endless generations will perish through the death of the pregnant."

Five hundred years later, persisting human compassion, reverence for motherhood, and zeal to improve the commonweal compel us to address this problem, for although we can now prevent most such disasters, some individual needless deaths continue. While losses are fewer, the pain and suffering of bereavement and orphanage are no less dreadful, and it is incumbent upon medicine and upon obstetrics in particular to keep a constant vigil lest the dark ages return.

HISTORY

In 1917 the New York Academy of Medicine, stimulated by an intolerable death rate in New York City, undertook the pioneer study which, after several intermissions, was finally published in 1933.[1] It not only engendered countless others but set an example of effective preventive medicine which, one notes with satisfaction, came from within the profession itself, did not rely upon government funding at any level, and was not motivated by the hope of partisan political advantage. The stringent and absolutely honest recommendations of that distinguished committee show organized medicine in action at its best.

At almost the same time, Dr. Philip Williams initiated in Philadelphia, a comparable but continuous study which was widely copied.[2] He was a giant in his day and perhaps more than any other single individual improved the lot of pregnant women in the United States.

The Obstetrical Society of Boston also began an investigation in 1933 of maternal mortality in the city of Boston.[3] Findings were so disturbing that, upon its urging, the Massachusetts Medical Society created a Committee on Maternal Welfare under the chairmanship of Robert deNormandie who began work in 1941.[4] Two hundred forty-seven deaths, discovered by inspection of death certificates in that one year, were studied in retrospect. World War II soon interrupted this, but in 1948 it was revived under the stimulus of Duncan E. Reid and a rejuvenated committee resumed the work which has now come to be recognized as an indispensable function of the society. Its work, under the chairmanship of Luke Gillespie, was reported in 1954.[5] Information included in this chapter is derived from the experience of the study from 1954 to 1983.

HOW THE STUDY OF MATERNAL MORTALITY IS CONDUCTED IN MASSACHUSETTS

This medical society's Committee on Maternal Welfare has been investigating maternal deaths for over four decades, during which the procedure has been refined. A description of our present protocol follows below, while certain terms are defined at the end of this chapter. This committee does not use the classification of direct obstetric, indirect obstetric, or nonrelated causes because we consider each death a medical failure from which something should be learned; the competent obstetrician treats every patient as a whole regardless of her problems. The renowned Frederick C. Irving once remarked that a pregnant woman is subject to the same diseases and conditions as any other woman with the sole exception of infertility.

Thanks to scrupulously observed guarantees of absolute confidentiality, voluntary individual reporting of maternal deaths has become normal practice. Although rules and regulations of the Department of Public Health require such reports from hospital administrators in writing within 48 hours, there is no penalty stipulated for failure to do so. The system of making voluntary reports directly to the committee has been found remarkably reliable; sometimes information is provided within an hour of the event. At the time, the reporting physician is urged to request a necropsy; the committee can provide assistance for such an examination when it might otherwise be impossible.

Probably the most important distinguishing feature of the Massachusetts study is the fact that a member of the committee interviews the responsible physician in person at a time convenient to them both. The prenatal record from clinic or office is reviewed and, with the physician's permission (which has never been denied), the hospital record is thoroughly studied. Further, a copy of the autopsy protocol and duplicate microscopic slides of the significant tissues are requested from the pathologist. Not infrequently the personal interview becomes highly informative to both parties; oversights or errors become clearly apparent in a sympathetic and objective review of the case history. We abjure the practice of submitting an impersonal (and usually inadequate) questionnaire for completion by the physician or an uninformed administrator.

Following collection of the available information, the case is reviewed by the assembled committee, at which time identity of the patient, physician, hospital, and community is concealed. Thus, reputations are sheltered and opinions are unbiased. The committee's pathologist presents independent interpretations of the postmortem findings, and the committee agrees upon a cause of death. Occasionally this is not identical with the one of record. After discussion, preventability is determined by majority vote and, if the death is deemed "preventable," a further vote is taken to assign responsibility. The assignee is usually the obstetrician or the patient. However, the family, a consultant, the anesthesiologist, the nursing staff, or the hospital administration may be chosen; some combination of these is occasionally appropriate. The substance of the discussion and the resulting opinion are then transmitted in detail to the responsible physician. No further report of this absolutely confidential information is rendered to anyone.

Although this study began before its records were protected from misuse in litigation, there exists now a statute in Massachusetts which, in effect, immunizes to subpoena all records, opinions, correspondence, and other files. The most important portion reads: "Such information, records, reports, statements, notes, memoranda, or other data shall not be admissible as evidence in any action of any kind in any court or before any other tribunal, board, agency, or person . . . " (Chapter 111, Section 24A of the General Laws of the Commonwealth of Massachusetts).[6] Thus far, that statute has not been challenged nor our efforts prostituted for private gain.

RESULTS OF A 30-YEAR STUDY IN MASSACHUSETTS

During the years 1954 through 1983, inclusive, there were 2,745,625 live births recorded in Massachusetts. In the same period 904 maternal deaths were reported to and studied by the committee. Without doubt some have escaped our attention, but the number not reported is thought to be very small. Any such cases later coming to light have been added to the data for each respective year.

Consistent with prevailing policy, these deaths have been classified according to "conditions" rather than "causes," there often being, in any given death, several contributory conditions, any one of which could not be considered the sole cause. Therefore, the total number of conditions, listed in order of frequency, exceeds the total number of deaths (Table 2-1).

Analysis

During the first seven years, the annual number of births in Massachusetts rose slowly, but thereafter it declined and now seems to have leveled off after a brief secondary rise. Concurrently the total number of deaths also diminished, as might be expected (Figure 2-1). However, the rate of diminution has far exceeded that of live births (Figure 2-2).

NCHS versus Massachusetts Medical Society Rates

It is apparent that there is underreporting of maternal deaths in this state by the National Center for Health Statistics (NCHS). As shown in Table 2-2 and Figure 2-3, for example, between 1964 and 1973, there were 136 deaths

Table 2-1
Conditions* Associated with Maternal Mortality, 1954–1983

Live births	2,745,625†
Maternal deaths	904
Hemorrhage	128
Sepsis	105
Toxemia	63
Heart disease	84
Intracranial accident	74
Pulmonary embolism	73
Disseminated intravascular coagulopathy	51
Malignancy	52
Septic shock	48
Anesthesia	48
Ruptured uterus	45
Renal failure	34
Amniotic fluid infusion	30
Intestinal obstruction	26
Drug related	22
Abruptio placentae	21
Pneumonia	21
Ectopic pregnancy	20
Viral pneumonitis	19
Diabetes mellitus	18
Miscellaneous conditions	80
Total conditions	1062
Cause of death undetermined	42
Total deaths	904

*Medical conditions only. Social, economic, and religious conditions were not the object of this study.
†Includes an estimated number of births in 1983.

reported by NCHS and 268 maternal deaths reported by the state committee. This disparity between maternal mortality rates reported by NCHS and local statistics has also been emphasized by the Centers for Disease Control and can be ascribed to a number of causes. First, maternal deaths may come to light locally after the total number has been conveyed to

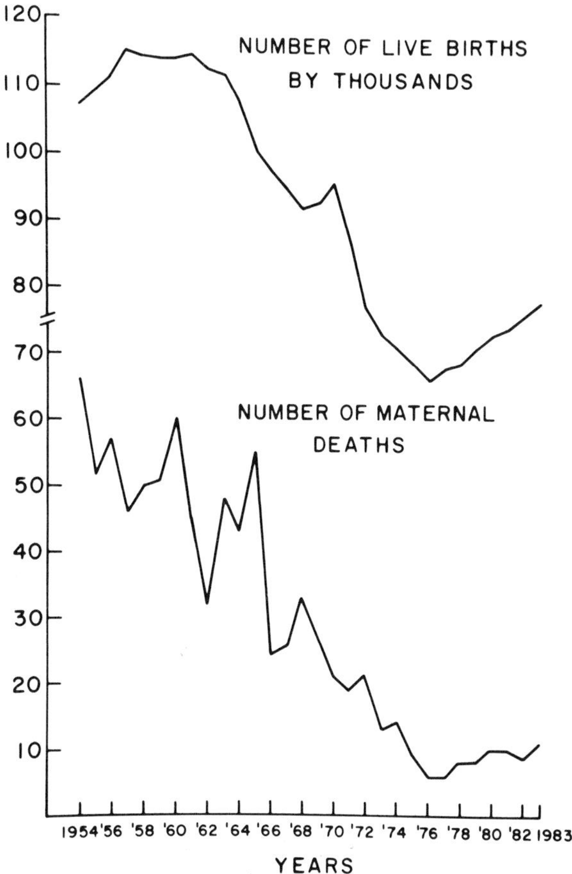

Figure 2-1 Number of live births and maternal deaths in Massachusetts, 1954–1983.

Washington. Second, divisions of vital statistics must depend on frequently inaccurate or incomplete death certificates, and in many states there is no requirement to indicate whether the female decedent has been recently pregnant. Lastly, the

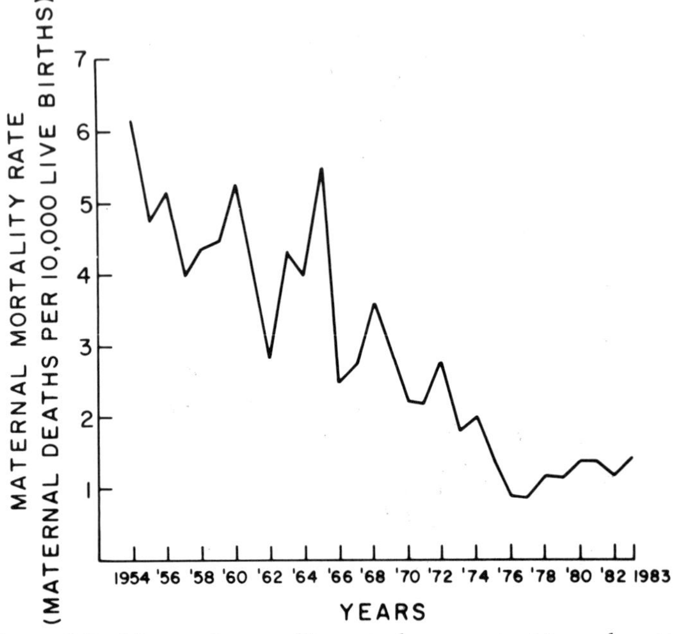

Figure 2-2 Maternal mortality rate by year in Massachusetts, 1954–1983.

Table 2-2
Number of Maternal Deaths Reported by NCHS and Massachusetts Maternal Welfare Committee

	NCHS	State committee
1941	247	247
1949–1953		194
1954–1963	238	502
1964–1973	136	268
1974–1983	22*	91

*1983 not available.

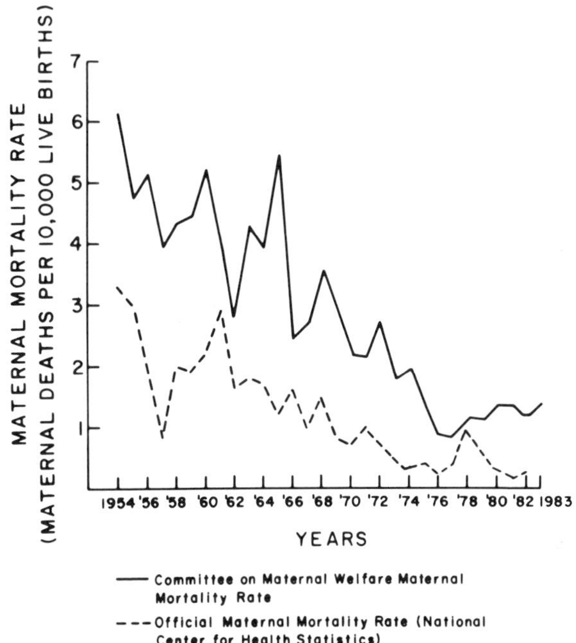

Figure 2-3 Comparison of NCHS and the Massachusetts Maternal Welfare Committee maternal mortality rates, 1954–1983.

definition of a maternal death may differ between the state committees and the NCHS, especially with respect to the number of inclusive days postpartum.

Causes of Death in Massachusetts

By any standard and by any definition, maternal welfare has been steadily enhanced in the United States. To see how much improvement has taken place during 30 years in Massachusetts, one can plot the frequency of those conditions comprising a triumvirate which has been recognized for

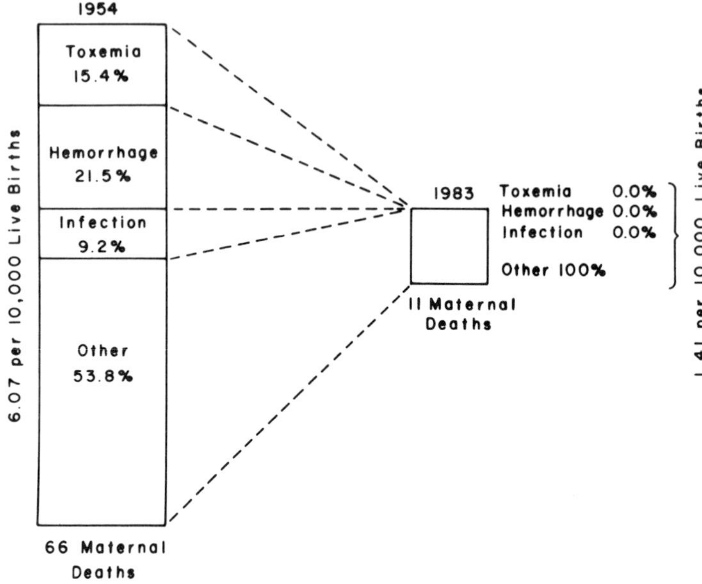

Figure 2-4 The classical triumvirate: causes of maternal mortality in Massachusetts, 1954–1983.

generations; namely, that of hemorrhage, infection, and toxemia (Figure 2-4). The temporary, but absolute, disappearance of one during 1973 and the eradication of all three in 1983 constitutes a justifiable source of self-congratulation by a profession which is far more accustomed to introspection and self-criticism. No doubt other factors than strictly medical ones have played a part in this extraordinary accomplishment, but that cannot dim our pride in having had an important part in it.

Another change has been the extraordinary difference in the general character of cases now demanding attention. In 1933 accouchment forcé, internal podalic version, high forceps operations, unnecessary cesarean sections, and raging sepsis combined to raise the price of reproduction. By con-

Table 2-3
Causes of Death*

Middlesex East District, 1882	State of Massachusetts, 1983
Puerperal peritonitis (4)	Homicide (1)
Embolism (3)	Adult respiratory distress syndrome (1)
Phthisis (2)	Acute myocardial infarction (1)
Puerperal septicemia (2)	Cerebral hemorrhage (1)
Chronic puerperal septicemia (1)	Subdural hematoma (1)
Erysipelas (1)	Viral myocarditis (1)
Puerperal convulsions (1)	Pheochromocytoma (1)
Postpartum hemorrhage (1)	Anesthetic accident/cardiac arrest (1)
Uremia (1)	Pulmonary embolus (1)
Renal disease (1)	Amniotic fluid embolism (1)
Rheumatic endocarditis (1)	Anesthetic accident/massive acute emphysema (unruptured ectopic pregnancy) (1)
Puerperal anemia (1)	

*Number of cases in parentheses.

trast, the variety of conditions lethal to only 11 women during 1983 among 77,500 live births make an even more fascinating contrast when compared to 19 deaths reported in 1882 among 2709 births[7] (Table 2-3). Very evidently the practice of obstetrics is one of general medicine which may involve every other specialty within the vocation.

Preventability

Considering that medicine has always been limited in its ability to correct the problems it meets, the categories of preventability yield perhaps the best criteria of success (Table 2-4). Unfortunately we cannot report a recognizable trend toward improvement in the proportion of preventable deaths among the totals. Figure 2-5 shows the relative frequency of

Table 2-4
30-Year Totals, 1954–1983 Inclusive

	Number	Percent
Preventable	322	35.6
Nonpreventable	444	49.1
Undetermined	138	15.3
Total	904	100

cases classified as preventable, nonpreventable, or undetermined, but the proportion of preventable deaths, as shown in Figure 2-6, has fluctuated between 50% and zero during these 30 years. Perhaps this phenomenon is attributable to the very low numbers in each category. It should be further pointed out that in many preventable cases, responsibility was assigned to the patient or her family. However, so long as

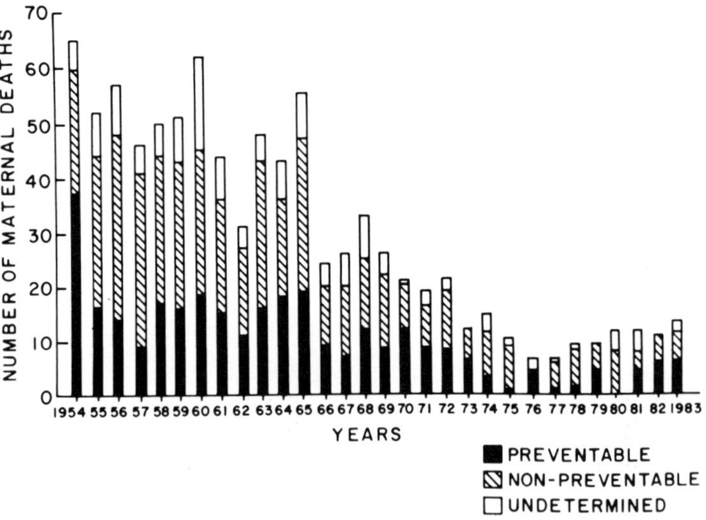

Figure 2-5 Frequency of preventable and nonpreventable maternal deaths in Massachusetts, 1954–1983.

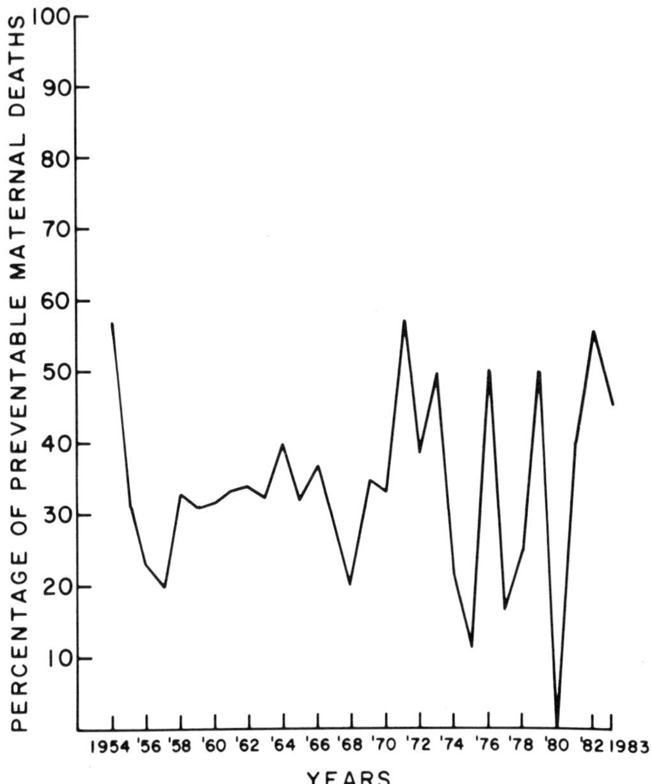

Figure 2-6 Percentage of preventable maternal deaths in Massachusetts, 1954–1983.

there remains one preventable death, we can never say that the maternal mortality rate is irreducible.

Use of Data

During this 30-year study, the primary motive has been one of education, while the practical application of statistics derived from it has been secondary, and there has been absolutely no place for a disciplinary role. The traditional concept of learning from our mistakes has dominated activities of the committee, whose members would be first to agree that their own individual benefits from its lessons have been incalculable.

A prime beneficiary is often the practitioner concerned. If, in our opinion, a given case has been marred by some medical error of commission or omission, the perpetrator is so informed by a studious, detailed, and objective dissertation on the points at issue. When an error stems from ignorance or mistaken judgement, education is paramount; the intent is to let the clinical lessons become evident to all concerned. Finally, of course, there are presumed educational benefits to the profession at large from cases chosen for publication.

It is impossible to measure all these presumed benefits. In fact, a serious attempt to do so was undertaken by Grimes and Cates at the Centers for Disease Control in 1977.[8] The maternal mortality rates in states with and without maternal death studies were determined. To our dismay, the rate of improvement did not correlate with the existence of such death studies. It seems likely, however, that the discrepancy lies in the assumption that mortality rates can be used as criteria for the efficacy of education; contributing and confounding factors are virtually innumerable.

Once used as a general yardstick to judge the quality of care in a given community or given hospital, the maternal mortality rate is now comprised of such small figures as to be invalid for this purpose. Nevertheless its overall general success has given rise to perinatal mortality studies which today are probably a far better index of a hospital's excellence.

Although secondary as a motive, practical uses have been made of the data in the past. A few examples can be cited: maternity units in Massachusetts are now limited to institutions with blood banks as a direct result of this committee's findings; minimum standards for obstetric care were drawn up and published largely because so many deaths resulted from inadequate prenatal care; regionalization of obstetric perinatal care was brought about largely because of maternal and perinatal mortality data.

Cesarean Section Mortality

The recent increase in use of cesarean section is universal and has been a source of concern to the profession.[9] It is not, as the lay press would have us believe, exclusively an American phenomenon nor is it socioeconomically related. Massachusetts did not require the registration of cesarean sections until 1976, and therefore firm figures for its frequency are not available until then. However, a recent retrospective audit was made by the Eastern Massachusetts Professional Standards Review Organization as part of a quality review study. All 26 hospitals with maternity units in this area reported their total figures for 15 years, yielding the composite data on its frequency shown in Figure 2-7. This is probably a fair representation of experience throughout the state, since about two thirds of the state's population reside in this area. Quite obviously the trend upward has reached a plateau; it is equally obvious that, despite the increased number of cesarean sections, there has been no increased number of maternal deaths.

Mortality of Cesarean Section versus Mortality of Vaginal Delivery

In Massachusetts between 1976 and 1981, the maternal mortality directly related to cesarean delivery was 1.63/10,000 operations. This compared to a maternal mortality of 0.78/10,000 deliveries following vaginal delivery. In order to understand how these data were derived, it is useful to look at the 21 deaths associated with cesarean delivery during

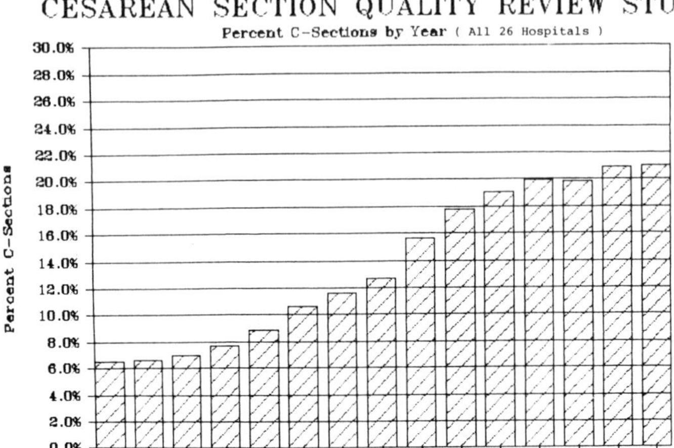

Figure 2-7 Cesarean section rates (26 hospitals) in Massachusetts, 1968–1982. Eastern Massachusetts Professional Standards Review Committee, unpublished data (1983).

those years, when there were 73,175 cesarean sections and 346,226 vaginal deliveries.

Nine of the 21 cases were discarded, including seven intra- and postmortem cesarean sections and two surgically unrelated. Since criteria of death and times of occurrence were not always clear in the hospital record and some operations were described as "agonal" or performed only pro forma to console the family, none were considered postmortem if the mother had perceptible vital signs recorded more than an hour afterward and unless it had been agreed preoperatively that maternal survival was utterly hopeless. There were two such cases, in both of which the infant was stillborn.

In addition, there were five cases best described as intramortem. So categorized were cases of women already in extremis from irreversibly fatal conditions but who survived the procedure by more than an hour because of life-support

Eastern College of Nursing Library

systems. These five deaths were caused by: advanced Crohn's disease with multiple bowel fistulae, carcinomatosis, decerebrate status following amniotic fluid embolus, massive intracranial hemorrhage, and acute fatty liver of pregnancy. In all of these, intervention was motivated by an attempt to obtain a living fetus before further maternal deterioration would cause brain damage to the infant. These five attempts yielded a living infant in all but one.

Finally, there were two cesarean sections performed because of congenital heart disease (Eisenmenger's syndrome). Both patients died on the fourth postpartum day as, in fact, did two other patients with the same heart condition who easily delivered vaginally. These deaths were considered unrelated to the surgery or the route of delivery. The infants did well.

These corrections thus left 12 deaths directly related to surgery, and we may conclude that the risk of a cesarean section is approximately twice the risk of a vaginal delivery in Massachusetts. This figure is consistent with the crude rate of cesarean section death versus overall maternal mortality at the Boston Hospital for Women in 25 years (Table 2-5). That record is superseded by the later experience of 11 years, with

Table 2-5
Six Studies Comparing Risks per 10,000 of Cesarean Section versus Vaginal Delivery

Evrard and Gold (RI)[11] 1965–1976	6.9 versus 0.27
Rubin et al (Georgia)[12] 1975–1977	5.9 versus 0.97
Massachusetts 1954–1975	4.9 versus 3.5 (overall)
Boston Hospital for Women 1954–1975	4.2 versus 2.00
Boston Hospital for Women[10] 1968–1978	0.0 versus 0.72
Massachusetts 1976–1981	1.63 versus 0.78

no maternal deaths among more than 10,000 cesarean deliveries reported at the same hospital by Frigoletto et al.[10]

Six different assessments of the risk of death at cesarean versus vaginal delivery are compared in Table 2-5.[10–12] Of note is the study in Georgia, conducted by the Centers for Disease Control, showing a sixfold higher risk.[12] All these deaths were directly due to the surgical procedure and not to a preexisting medical condition, using the same method of case analysis we used in Massachusetts. This difference in reported risks may reflect the earlier time of the study as well as disparate patient populations.

Cesarean Section: Risks and Benefits for Mother and Fetus

The increased frequency of cesarean section over the last decade has resulted largely from an attempt to improve fetal outcome, but its impact on maternal health has not been adequately addressed. For example, many academic studies advocate cesarean delivery for breech presentation and as an alternative to a difficult forceps operation. Practices that ensued from these recommendations have become standard, with smaller, less well-equipped hospitals forced to follow suit. One would expect larger teaching institutions to accommodate a rise in the number of cesarean sections as their facilities can provide adequate anesthesia coverage, blood banking, and all the other factors that enhance the safety of surgery. However, this may not be true for smaller institutions, particularly with respect to anesthesia. Thus, if mortality and morbidity related to cesarean section is higher in smaller institutions than in teaching institutions, then risks and benefits for mother and fetus will differ according to where the obstetrical care is being delivered. We postulate that this is so.

Only one study has examined this issue on the basis of population. Under the aegis of the Centers for Disease Control in Atlanta,[13] this study chose as an example the issues of breech presentations and low-birth-weight infants in cephalic presentations. Showing first that infants presenting by the breech and certain categories of infants with normal presentations but of low birth weight will benefit from cesarean delivery, the authors went on to calculate what would have been the expected rise in maternal mortality related to cesarean section if these infants had been delivered by cesarean section.

Computer-linked birth and infant-death records from the Georgia Neonatal Surveillance System were used. There were 392,241 singleton deliveries from 1974 through 1978, and in this five-year period there were 9626 singleton breech deliveries (2%); of these newborns, 1793 (19%) weighed 2500 g or less. In addition, there were 25,589 singleton vertex deliveries with a recorded birth weight of 2500 g or less. Among all these births, the risk of neonatal death for breech infants weighing 1000–4000 g was significantly greater for those delivered vaginally than those delivered by cesarean section. For high-risk infants in cephalic presentation weighing 1000–1500 g, the lowest neonatal mortality rate occurred among those delivered by cesarean section and managed in a tertiary perinatal center. Although these results do not indicate that all low-birth-weight infants should be delivered by cesarean section, they strongly suggest that in complicated pregnancies (eg, hypertension, infection, or antepartum hemorrhage), when the infant can be expected to weigh 1000–1500 g, the mother should be treated in, or transferred to, a tertiary perinatal unit and the infant delivered by cesarean section.

Finally, the authors examined the expected effect in Georgia of performing cesarean sections for breech infants weighing 1000–2500 g and for high-risk vertex infants weighing 1000–1500 g. If all such infants had been delivered by cesarean section, they estimated that an additional 5206 operations (17% increase) would have had to be performed to save 172 infants, of which 133 would have been low birth weight, thus requiring specialized neonatal care. Furthermore, using an excess maternal mortality rate of 4.96/10,000 cesarean sections,[12] three additional maternal deaths would have occurred. An estimate of the increased financial cost of performing the additional 5206 sections in Georgia over five years and the support of 133 low-birth-weight infants in intensive care units was $8.76 million. Maternal morbidity related to cesarean section includes: (1) a 7- to 20-fold increase in maternal infection, (2) increased length of hospital stay, (3) longer convalescence, and (4) the psychological effect of major surgery. In addition, many of the women would have required a later repeat cesarean section since the uterine incision for premature breech is frequently vertical. Not meant to be a cost–benefit analysis, especially as some of the variables were unknown, the results simply underline the maternal costs of cesarean section.

The authors conclude that if neonatal morbidity can be shown to decline significantly as a result of more frequent cesarean sections, the benefits may outweigh the costs; however, this will require further study. The increase in maternal risks from increasing the cesarean section rate, for indications discussed, is small, but it may vary between institutions. In those institutions where the maternal risk of surgery is higher, the obstetrician and the patient must accept either limited indications for cesarean section or maternal transport to a tertiary perinatal center.

REPRODUCTIVE MORTALITY

Maternal mortality has declined in the United States by 50% during the last decade.[14] The decline has coincided with an increase in the use of contraception, sterilization, and legal abortion. A survey reported by the National Center for Health Statistics showed that 22% of women aged 15–44 used oral contraceptives.[15] To examine the consequences of these

Table 2-6
Components of Reproductive Mortality

Pregnancy related
Ectopic
Abortion spontaneous/induced
All other pregnancy-related causes
Contraception related
Oral contraception
Intrauterine devices
Sterilization

changes, Beral proposed the use of the reproductive mortality rate (RMR) as a measure of the hazards of fertility and fertility control.[16]

This rate includes deaths due to the adverse effects of temporary contraceptive methods and of sterilization as well as maternal deaths. Beral defined the latter as deaths due to ectopic pregnancies, spontaneous and induced abortions, and all other pregnancy-related deaths (Table 2-6). Deaths due to induced abortion might be attributed more appropriately to fertility control rather than pregnancy. However, only since the liberalization of abortion laws has it been possible to separate deaths due to induced abortion from those due to spontaneous abortion and thus, in recent years at least, induced-abortion-related deaths account for only a small proportion of maternal deaths. Beral reported for England and Wales that the reproductive mortality rate declined steadily after 1950 for women aged 25–34 years. For women aged 35–44 years, however, the reproductive mortality rate increased after 1960 because of the relatively higher mortality rate associated with oral contraception in this age group.

Reproductive Mortality in the United States

In a similar study conducted by the Centers for Disease Control, estimates were made of reproductive mortality in

Table 2-7
Age-Specific Reproductive Mortality in the United States: 1955, 1965, and 1975

Year and age group	Reproductive mortality rate*
1955	
15–19	4.0
20–34	9.8
34–44	6.4
Total	7.8
1965	
15–19	2.0
20–34	6.1
35–44	5.7
Total	5.1
1975	
15–19	0.8
20–34	1.9
35–44	3.8
Total	2.1

*Rate per 100,000 women.

the United States for 1955, 1965, and 1975. Results were derived from the best available data on pregnancy-related mortality, contraception-related mortality, and the prevalence of various contraceptive practices.[17]

Between 1955 and 1975, the estimated RMR in the United States fell by 73% among women aged 15–44 years from 7.8/100,000 in 1955 to 2.1 in 1975 (Table 2-7). The decrease was greater for women younger than 35; for women aged 15–34 years, the rate fell by about 80%, but for those aged 35–44 years it fell by 41% during the 20-year period.

In 1955, 99% of reproductive deaths were pregnancy-related, in contrast to 53% in 1975 (Figure 2-8). In 1955, prior to the advent of oral contraception and intrauterine devices, less than 1% of reproductive deaths were related to contraception (all due to sterilization); however, 15% in 1965, and 47%

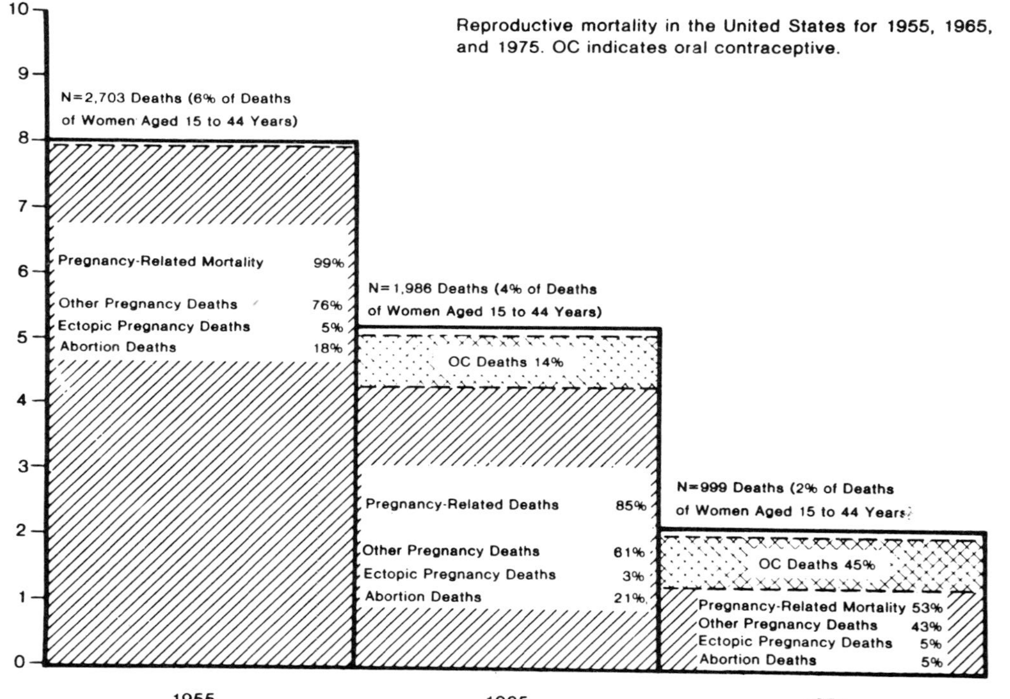

Figure 2-8 Reproductive mortality in the United States[17] for 1955, 1965, and 1975. OC indicates oral contraceptive.

in 1975, were due to contraception and sterilization. Oral contraception (OC) in 1975 was responsible for 45% of the deaths. Obviously, the relative importance of the various components of reproductive mortality had changed markedly those two decades. Pregnancy-related mortality declined rapidly (86%), while contraceptive mortality and, in particular, OC-related deaths increased. The smaller decline in the RMR (41%) for women aged 35–44 years was due primarily to deaths from oral contraception. In this older group there were almost 350 deaths due to OC usage.

Reproductive Mortality in Massachusetts

It has been recommended that surveillance of maternal mortality be expanded to include all reproductive deaths. Under the auspices of the Massachusetts Medical Society's Committee on Maternal Welfare and the Division of Family Health Services of the commonwealth's Department of Public Health, an investigation of reproductive deaths in Massachusetts was conducted for 1981.[18]

Method As described above, the Committee on Maternal Welfare identifies pregnancy-related deaths and, by the time this study was conducted, had already completed its review of those in 1981. The contraception-related deaths were identified as follows: 11 codes from the ninth revision of the International Classification of Diseases were selected as potential indicators of complications due to fertility control. All death certificates with these codes were retrieved by the Department of Public Health. In most cases the cause of death had been confirmed by autopsy, and those that could not be classified as reproductive deaths were discarded. All the remaining cases were investigated. This investigation included a review of hospital records and, when available, findings at autopsy. In selected cases, the medical examiner or the primary physician or both were interviewed. Deaths were classified as not related, unlikely, or probably related to contraceptives.

Results Fourteen reproductive deaths were identified in 1981. Four of them were due to pregnancy prevention. Three of these were considered preventable because, in each, oral contraception was contraindicated, as all three were known to be hypertensive and over the age of 35; two were also smokers. The Committee on Maternal Welfare had reported eight pregnancy-related deaths in 1981. This study discovered two more, resulting in a maternal mortality rate of 1.3/10,000 live births. The committee had decided that four of these maternal deaths were preventable. The overall RMR was 1.9/10,000 live births (1/100,000 women, Table 2-8). For women aged 15–34, one out of the nine deaths was related to oral contraceptives. For women aged 35–44, three out of the five deaths were related to oral contraceptives.

Oral contraceptive mortality rates in Massachusetts The Division of Preventive Medicine of the Department of Public Health in 1980 surveyed the health-related behavior

Table 2-8
Mortality among Massachusetts Women in Relation to Pregnancy, Smoking, and Oral Contraception, According to Age Group*

	Mortality rate			
		Contraceptive related deaths‡		
Age group	*Pregnancy-related deaths*†	Smokers	Nonsmokers	*RMR*§
15–34	0.8	0.8	0	0.9
34–44	0.6	25.8	8.6	1.5
15–44	0.7	2.4	0.8	1.0

*Massachusetts Department of Public Health Survey, 1980.[22]
†Deaths per 100,000 women.
‡Deaths per 100,000 users of oral contraceptives.
§Reproductive mortality rate (deaths per 100,000 women).

of 1091 adults in Massachusetts. This survey showed that 23% of women under the age of 35 used oral contraception and that 50% of this group were smokers. For women aged 35–44, only 6% were users of oral contraception but 40% of them were smokers. The at-risk population was calculated by using these figures and applying them to the number of women in Massachusetts in each age group as determined by the 1980 national census. Thus, the estimated mortality rates associated with oral contraception are as follows: 0.8/100,000 users for women aged 15–34 and 15.5/100,000 users for women aged 35–44 (Table 2-8). For women over 35 who smoke, however, the mortality rate associated with oral contraception rises dramatically to 26/100,000 users. Because of the small numbers, these mortality rates must be considered estimates of the risk of oral contraception.

CONCLUSIONS

Oral contraceptives are very safe for the majority of women. The reproductive mortality rate is a better criterion than the maternal mortality rate for measuring the risks of reproduction in an era of low fertility. The overall RMR in Massachusetts is very low: 1/100,000 women. In 1981 the number of preventable pregnancy-related deaths was almost the same as the number of preventable oral-contraception-related deaths. Deaths due to pregnancy prevention were confined to oral contraception, the risk of which was very small for women under 35. However, the risks of oral contraception were higher than those of pregnancy for women over the age of 35. Further improvement in the reproductive mortality rate could be achieved by proscribing the pill for women over 35 and especially for smokers or hypertensive women.

"Mothers are still mortal."[19] Although maternal mortality has been reduced dramatically in the United States and less dramatically elsewhere in the past 30 years, there is evident room for improvement. So long as a single preventable death occurs, the rate is not irreducible and efforts for surveillance must therefore continue. Continuing education of physicians and the reeducation of the public are paramount. Equally important is use of the data by experts in public health to reveal geographic, social, and economic factors amenable to improvement.

DEFINITIONS

For the purposes of this chapter the following definitions apply:

Maternal death A maternal death is the death of a woman while pregnant or during a stated period of time following pregnancy. (Most surveys limit this period to 90 days, some to six weeks, and a few extend this time to one full year.) It should be emphasized at the outset that "maternal deaths" so defined bear only a remote relation to those reported by the various bureaus or divisions of vital statistics, whose duty it is to record those deaths due to causes coded by the ICDA-9 under rubrics numbered 640–676.[20]

Maternal mortality rate The number of deaths in a given time is customarily compared to the number of live births in the same time period. More accurately this is called a maternal mortality ratio. Ideally the denominator should be the total number of pregnancies, but the latter is neither officially recorded nor otherwise available and estimates are inaccurate at best.

Direct obstetric cause of death A death resulting from complications of the pregnancy itself, from intervention elected or required by the pregnancy, or resulting from the chain of events initiated by the complication or the intervention.[21]

Indirect obstetric cause of death A death resulting from disease before or developing during pregnancy (not a direct effect of the pregnancy) which was obviously aggravated by the physiological effects of the pregnancy and caused the death.[21]

Nonobstetric cause of death A death occurring during pregnancy or within 90 days of its termination from causes not related to pregnancy or to its complications or management.[21]

Preventable death A death is considered preventable if, with other medical management, the patient would have survived; included also are deaths in which the patient, her family, or others responsible failed to follow instructions, refused treatment, delayed medical attention, or otherwise interfered with proper care.

Nonpreventable death Nonpreventable deaths are those in which there has been no demonstrable critical error of commission or omission on the part of anyone involved. General and nonmedical considerations are avoided, such as the hypothetical preventability of automobile accidents and homicides.

Undetermined preventability When the cause of death cannot be determined, preventability cannot be determined. Thus the lack of any autopsy often demands this type of classification. The same applies when the disease process is so severe that success of any management is in question even if there are evident deficiencies in treatment.

REFERENCES

1. Hooker RS: *Maternal Mortality in New York City: A Study of All Puerperal Deaths 1930–1932.* New York, Oxford University Press, 1933.
2. Williams PF: *Maternal Mortality in Philadelphia, 1931–1933.* Committee on Maternal Welfare of the Philadelphia County Medical Society, (Reported in 1934).
3. De Normandie RL, et al: Maternity mortality in Boston for the years 1933,1934,1935: Study conducted by the Obstetrical Society of Boston and the Department of Public Health. *N Engl J Med* 1937;216:43–51.
4. Massachusetts Medical Society: Analysis of causes of maternal death in Massachusetts during 1941. *N Engl J Med* 1942;227:611,

650, 685, 722, 807, 850–852, 889, 935, 972, 1008–1011, 1054–1056. *N Engl J Med* 1943;228:36, 78, 109, 141, 172, 205, 266.
5. Gillespie L: Maternal deaths in Massachusetts. *Trans N Engl Obstet Gynecol Soc* 1954;8:53–59.
6. Editorial. In defense of scientific studies. *N Engl J Med* 1960;263:974.
7. Abbott SW: Summary of obstetric cases. *Boston Med Surg J* 1882; 107:3–6.
8. Grimes DA, Cates W Jr: The impact of maternal mortality study committees on maternal deaths in the United States. *Am J Public Health* 1977;67(9):830–833.
9. Bottoms SF, Rosen MG, Sokol RJ: The increase in the cesarean birth rate. *N Engl J Med* 1980;302:559–563.
10. Frigoletto FD Jr, Ryan KJ, Phillippe M: Maternal mortality associated with cesarean section: An appraisal. *Am J Obstet Gynecol* 1980;136:969–970.
11. Evrard JR, Gold EM: Cesarean section and maternal mortality in Rhode Island. *Obstet Gynecol* 1977;50:594–597.
12. Rubin GL, Peterson HB, Rochat RW, et al: Maternal death after cesarean section in Georgia. *Am J Obstet Gynecol* 1981;139(6): 681–685.
13. Sachs BP, McCarthy BJ, Rubin G, et al: Cesarean section: Risks and benefits for mother and fetus. *JAMA* 1983;250:2157–2159.
14. Rochat RW: Maternal mortality in the United States of America. *World Health Stat Q* 1981;34:2–13.
15. National Center of Health Statistics: *Contraceptive Utilization in the United States: 1973.* 1976, Advance data No 36, August 1978.
16. Beral V: Reproductive mortality. *Br Med J* 1979;2:632–634.
17. Sachs BP, Layde PM, Rubin GL, et al: Reproductive mortality in the United States. *JAMA* 1982;247:2789–2792.
18. Sachs BP, Masterson T, Jewett JF, et al: Reproductive mortality in Massachusetts in 1981. *N Engl J Med* 1984;311:667–670.
19. Hofmeister FJ: Mothers are still mortal. *South Med J* 1978;71: 1193–1196.
20. Commission on Professional and Hospital Activities: *The International Classification of Diseases, 9th Revision, Clinical Modification.* Ann Arbor, MI, Edwards Brothers, 1978.
21. Council on Medical Service: *A Guide for Maternal Death Studies.* Chicago, American Medical Association, 1964.
22. Lambert CA, Netherton DR, Finision LJ, et al: Risk factors and life style: A statewide health-interview survey. *N Engl J Med* 1982;306:1048–51.

CHAPTER 3

EPIDEMIOLOGY OF PRETERM BIRTH

Phillip G. Stubblefield, MD

DEFINING THE PROBLEM

Premature delivery and low birth weight are the central issues in perinatal health care. In 1979, 17% of all births in the world were low birth weight. These accounted for 75% or more of the neonatal and infant deaths in the world.[1] Premature means born too early. The probability that an infant will survive is very strongly determined by gestational age at birth and increases from zero probability of survival at 22–23 weeks from the onset of the mother's last menstrual period, to almost certain survival by 40 menstrual weeks, full term. Survival after birth at 37 weeks is almost as likely as survival after full-term birth, and by convention, premature is defined as birth prior to 37 menstrual weeks (less than 259 days from the first day of the last menstrual period).[1]

Establishing the length of gestation can be difficult. In general, the single best criterion is the first day of the last normal menstrual period. However, there is variation in womens' ability to recall the date of the last menses, variation in the length of time from last menses to the ovulation that led to pregnancy, and sometimes early pregnancy bleeding confuses the issue. For the majority of women menstrual data is accurate and leads to the best estimate of length of gestation; however, for some pregnancies, use of menstrual data alone leads to considerable inaccuracy in determining the length of gestation. With the best of modern technology, ultrasound measurement of fetal size, a good estimate of gestational age is possible, provided the ultrasound measurements are taken in mid-pregnancy; even then, variations in rates of growth in utero make dating of pregnancy accurate only within a range of plus or minus 11 days.[2] Gestation can be dated exactly provided the woman has been measuring her basal body temperature daily during the cycle in which conception occurred. This allows dating of gestation from the day of ovulation. When this is done, the variation in average length of gestation becomes much less. Because of the difficulties in easily determining gestational age, birth weight has been used instead as a measure of fetal maturity.

In general, the correspondence between gestational age and birth weight is close[3] (Figure 3-1). By convention low birth weight is defined as weight less than 2500 g, and this is used as an equivalent for prematurity. Very low birth weight is taken to mean weight less than 1500 g at birth. Although low weight at birth is customarily used as equivalent to premature, this usage obscures part of the problem. Babies weighing more than 2500 g may be born before 37 weeks. In fact, in a sea level data set from the United States (Figure 3-1), half of babies born at 35 weeks weigh more than 2500 g.[3] By a weight definition, they would not be considered premature, an obvious mistake. Similarly, using 2500 g as the definition of low birth weight is not truly accurate for a US birth set. The 10th percentile is the usual criterion for pathologic "intrauterine growth retardation" or "IUGR." The 10th percentile at 40 weeks in a sea level data set is 2750 g, and infants weighing more than 2500 g but less the 2750 g should also be considered as low birth weight.

Although birth weight and gestational age are very highly correlated, they do not correspond exactly. The relationship

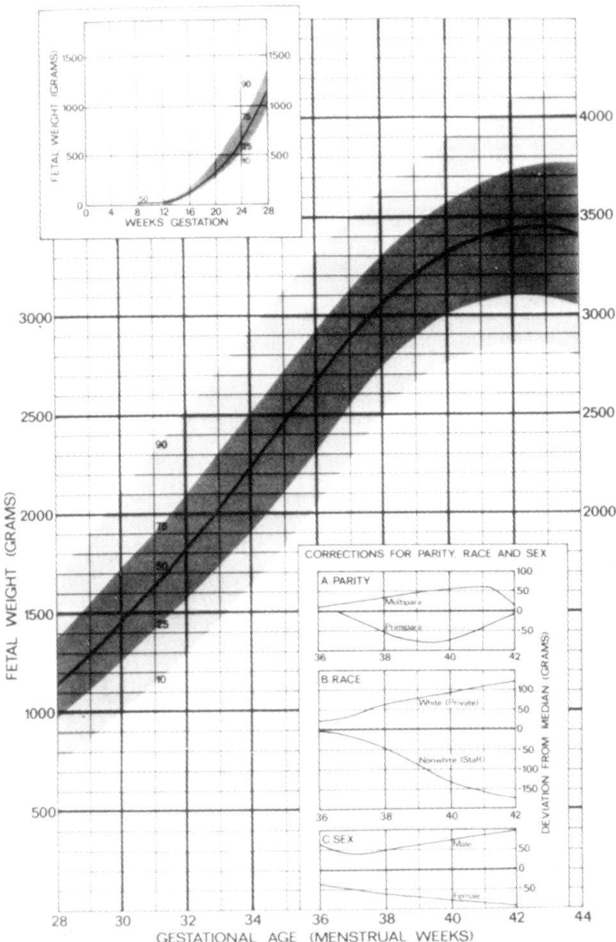

Figure 3-1 Fetal weight. The 50th (median), 10th, 25th, 75th, and 90th percentiles of fetal weight in grams throughout pregnancy and correction factors for parity, race (socioeconomic), and sex derived from 31,202 prostaglandin-induced abortions and "spontaneous" deliveries. Source: Brenner WE, Edelman DA, Hendricks CH: A standard of fetal growth for the United States of America. *Am J Obstet Gynecol* 1976;126:555–564,[3] by permission.

between either parameter and survival is a continuum. As birth weight or gestational age increases, chance of survival increases until average birth weight or in the case of gestational age, 37 weeks, is reached. There is no sudden improvement in survival when 2500 g is reach by comparison with 2400 g, or 37 weeks as compared with 36. In general, within birth weight groups, infants of more advanced gestational ages are more likely to survive, and within gestational age groups, the larger infants do better. Most attempts to study causes of low birth weight and prematurity have grouped births in large categories and compare all infants weighing less than 2500 g to those weighing more. This simple univariate grouping includes both true prematures and term low-birth-weight infants in the same group, a simplification that may well obscure causation of these separate but related problems.

Yerushalmy proposed a bivariate classification using both birth weight and gestational age, thus generating five groups[4] (Table 3-1). Other schemes, still more complicated, have been made. The most sophisticated is that of Hoffman et al: a contour map connecting gestational age and birthweight.[5] As a simple compromise for description of large data sets, one can separate preterm low birth weight (defined as born before 37 weeks and weighing less than 2500 g) from

Table 3-1
Suggested "Five-Group" Classification of Newborn Infants by Birth Weight and Gestational Age*

Group	Birth weight (g)	Gestation (weeks)
I	1500 or less	All gestations
II	1501–2500	Less than 37
III	1501–2500	37 or more
IV	2501 or more	Less than 37
V	2501 or more	37 or more

*Source: Yerushalmy, p 116,[4] by permission.

term low birth weight (defined as born at or after 37 weeks and weighing less than 2500 g).[4] In a key article, Villar and Belizan studied a number of international data sets containing both birth weight and gestational age.[6] They noted that in developing countries where the incidence of low birth weight (LBW) is generally very high, most of the LBW infants are born after 37 weeks, ie, they are growth retarded rather than premature. In the developed countries, the rate of LBW is much lower, less then 10%, and more of the LBW infants are true prematures.

LOW BIRTH WEIGHT AND PERINATAL MORTALITY

Most of the difference between countries in perinatal and infant mortality is accounted for by the differences in birth weight.[7] Sweden has the lowest proportion of LBW in the world, 3.6% in 1973, and the lowest national perinatal mortality rate in the world, 5 per 1000.[1] Mathematical adjustment of death rates to reflect different birth-weight distributions can offer insights into the causes of the deaths. Guyer and colleagues note that while neonatal mortality for the state of Massachusetts is higher than that of Sweden, the proportion of low birth weight (LBW) infants born is considerably greater here.[8] In fact, individual LBW infants are more likely to survive in Massachusetts than in Sweden, because of our neonatal intensive care units. When Massachusetts mortality statistics are adjusted to the Swedish birth-weight distribution, the calculated mortality rates for Massachusetts become less than those of Sweden. This statistical manipulation saves no lives, but does help clarify the issue: our incidence of low birth weight is the problem.

CAUSES OF LOW BIRTH WEIGHT

Most studies of the causes of prematurity have used a birth weight definition and are therefore studies of the associations of fetal growth retardation as well as short gestation. A large number of variables have been found as significantly related to the incidence of low birth weight.

Multiple Gestation

Average birth weights are greatest for singleton pregnancies; as the number of gestations increases to twins, triplets, and beyond, average birth weights decrease and risk of low birth weight increases. This phenomenon presumably is the result of limitations in the mother's ability to supply sufficient nutrients for optimum growth of more than one fetus. Because of the very marked effect of multiple gestations on weight at birth, studies of prematurity have usually excluded twins.

Mother's Size

Reciprocal crosses between large and small breeds of rabbits or horses show that the mother's size determines size of offspring. If the mare is of a large breed, the colt will be large.[9] In human populations, the mother's size is very important. As maternal prepregnant weight increases, average birth weight increases and risk of low birth weight decreases. For US data, average birth weight increases and risk of low birth weight decreases with increasing maternal height up to 66 inches, after which there is no further increase.[10] Of course, weight and height are associated, and all of the variation in birth weight by maternal height is said to be accounted for by maternal weight differences.[11]

Maternal Nutrition in Pregnancy

A multivariate analysis of birth weight and related factors among multiparous women found maternal weight gain during pregnancy to be the single most important determinant of birth weight.[10] Maternal weight gain in pregnancy profoundly affects infant birth weight, independent of maternal size. In areas where malnutrition is common, rates of low birth weight are very high. Proportions of LBW as high as 48% are reported from highland Guatemalan Indian villages with endemic malnutrition.[9] When women in late pregnancy are exposed to starvation, the effects on the pregnancy are devastating. Susser and Stein studied the effects on pregnancy of the famine in Holland at the end of World War II. Birth weight fell dramatically and neonatal mortality increased markedly for infants exposed to famine in the third trimester of pregnancy.[12]

Genetic Factors

Individuals who have produced one low-birth-weight or premature infant are highly likely to produce another subsequently,[13] but in the individual case it is rarely possible to separate what may be environmental factors from genetic ones. On the other hand, race and ethnicity furnish a crude segregation of human populations with genetic differences, and race does not affect birth weight and incidence of low birth weight. Comparison of black and white races in the United States show somewhat larger birth weight for black infants born prior to 34 menstrual weeks, but lower birth weights after that point, and the rates of low birth weight are approximately twice as high for black infants as for white infants (Table 3-2). The black average birth weight in the United States is about 200 g less than the white, and the average length of gestation is 9 days shorter for blacks.[10] The extent to which these differences are the result of genetic variation as opposed to the many social factors, for which race is but a convenient marker, is not known. However, an effect of race can be found even after attempting to control for such social and individual factors as income, education, occupation, and

Table 3-2
Percent of Live Births with Low Birth Weight* by Age of Mother and Race: United States 1970, 1975, and 1979†

	All races‡			White			Black		
Age of mother	*1979*	*1975*	*1970*	*1979*	*1975*	*1970*	*1979*	*1975*	*1970*
All ages	6.9	7.4	7.9	5.8	6.3	6.8	12.6	13.1	13.9
Under 15 years	14.5	14.1	16.6	11.8	11.3	12.5	16.7	16.2	19.1
15–19 years	9.6	10.0	10.5	7.9	8.1	8.6	14.2	14.8	15.7
20–24 years	7.0	7.1	7.4	5.8	6.0	6.4	12.5	12.8	13.4
25–29 years	5.9	6.1	6.9	5.1	5.4	6.2	11.2	11.2	12.2
30–34 years	5.9	6.8	7.5	5.2	6.1	6.7	11.3	11.8	12.3
35–39 years	7.4	8.2	8.7	6.5	7.3	7.8	12.2	13.2	13.4
40 and over	8.6	9.5	9.2	7.6	8.7	8.4	12.6	13.0	12.9

*Low birth weight is defined as less than 2500 g for 1979, and 2500 g or less for prior years.
†Source: Ventura SJ: Trends in first births to older mothers, 1970–1979. *Monthly Vital Statistics Report*. 31(2):Supp. 2, May 27, 1982, p 13, by permission.
‡Includes races other than white and black.

cigarette smoking. In a New York data set, incidence of low birth weight was greatest among blacks, least among whites, and intermediate for Hispanics.[14]

Maternal Age, Birth Order

Average birth weight increases progressively with maternal age,[10] but rates of low birth weight are highest for the youngest mothers, least for mothers aged 25–34 in the United States, and then increase with increasing maternal age thereafter (Table 3-2). Within the group of young mothers, a further refinement in predicting risk is the calculation of "gynecologic age," the number of years since menarche. In Zlatnik and Burmeister's study from Ohio, young adolescents who were two years or less from menarche when their infants were born had higher rates of low birth weight than girls of the same chronologic age but greater gynecologic age.[15]

The interaction of both variables, maternal age and birth order, is critical. In general, second or third births are less likely to be low birth weight than are first births. However, Puffer and Serrano discovered several years ago that second births to mothers under 20 are at much greater risk of low birth weight and infant mortality than first births, and third births to mothers under 20 are at even greater risk.[16] In order for a woman under 20 to have three births, the interval between pregnancies must be short, and short birth interval appears to independently increase risk of low birth weight. The original data were not adjusted in any way for social class, prenatal care, or any other such variables that might affect the outcome. However, Puffer and Serrano's study, although using primarily data from Latin America, included data sets from California and Canada where the same observation held true even though the magnitude of risk was less: higher-order births to mothers under 20 were at great risk of infant mortality associated with immaturity and low birth weight. This association has been found wherever it has been looked for.

Interpregnancy Interval

Short intervals are associated with low birth weight and high perinatal mortality, but this is also a tautology: short intervals from one birth to the next also include second births after short gestations, which of course means low birth weight. As recently analyzed by Winikoff, much of this data is badly confounded; however, very short intervals from birth to conception (less than six months or less than four months) are persistently associated with poorer outcomes in the next pregnancy.[17] One of the best of these studies is that of Fedrick and Adelstein. When the interval from birth to the next calculated time of conception was less than six months, there was excess of both low birth weight and true prematurity after controlling for maternal age and socioeconomic status.[18]

Altitude

As altitude increases, mean birth weight decreases, and frequency of low birth weight increases.[19] The reason for this is presumed to be the decreased oxygen tension of higher altitudes which limits the mother's ability to supply oxygen to the fetus. The increase in low birth weight at high altitudes reflects slower growth in utero rather than shorter gestation.

Maternal Illness

Illness that involves the circulatory system may contribute to low birth weight if severe. Among these are juvenile diabetes mellitus, chronic hypertension, chronic renal disease, cyanotic heart disease, and lupus erythematosis. These illnesses, fortunately, are very uncommon among women of childbearing age and make little contribution to the overall problem of low birth weight. Niswander reports association between low birth weight and bronchial asthma, hyperthyroidism, glomerulonephritis, urinary infections with a temperature of 100.4°F or higher, appendicitis, and organic heart disease.[20] The detailed analysis of data from the Collaborative Perinatal Project by Friedman and Neff found increasing rates of low birth weight as maternal diastolic blood pressure increased.[21] Within groups with similar blood pressures, low birth weight increased as proteinuria increased.

Cervical Incompetence

Cervical dilatation occurring in the mid-trimester with no apparent uterine contractions is termed incompetent cervix. The cause is generally unknown, but some cases are the result of previous cervical injury as with late induced abortion or extensive cone biopsy of the cervix. Cervical incompetence can be successfully treated by placement of a cerclage suture around the cervical opening. The availability of a treatment has contributed to frequent overdiagnosing of the condition in some areas.[22]

Maternal Infections

Many specific infectious diseases are associated with low birth weight or short gestation. These have been recently expertly reviewed by Polk and are summarized in Table 3-3.[23] In addition to these specific conditions, there is growing evidence that a number of different microorganisms that regularly colonize the vagina and cervix may at times be capable of producing an ascending infection of the fetal membranes that can reduce fetal growth and provoke preterm labor. Several years ago, Driscoll pointed out that placental inflammation, or "chorioamnionitis" was found in 50% of placentae from infants weighing less than 1000 g, and in 20% of placentae from infants weighing less than 2500 g, but in only 11% of all placentae.[24] Naeye and Peters found amniotic fluid infection syndrome to be the major cause of

Table 3-3
Specific Infections Associated with Low Birth Weight or Premature Delivery*

Condition	Low birth weight	Prematurity
Protozoal infections		
Malaria	+	+
Toxoplasmosis	+	+
Bacterial infections		
Syphilis	+	+
Tuberculosis		+
Leprosy		+
Typhoid fever		+
Listeriosis		+
Campylobacter		+
Suprative pelvic infections, eg, salpingitis or appendicitis		+
Urinary tract infections	+	+
Viral infections		
Infectious hepatitis		+
Measles		+
Smallpox		+
Rubella	+	
Cytomegalovirus	+	
Herpes simplex		+

*Source: Polk BF: Infectious processes and preterm labor, in Fuchs F, Stubblefield PG (eds): *Preterm Birth: Causes, Prevention and Management*. New York, Macmillan, 1984, pp 86–97, by permission.

perinatal mortality in the large US collaborative study.[25] In this syndrome fetal membranes were intact at onset of labor, and yet there was histologic evidence of placental inflammation consistent with infection.

Another line of evidence for an association between infection and low birth weight was provided by Elder and colleagues in Boston.[26] They performed a randomized trial of tetracycline versus placebo in bacteriuric and nonbacteriuric women to test their observation that bacteriuria was associated with low birth weight. Surprisingly, the nonbacteriuric women treated with tetracycline also had fewer preterm deliveries than control. Tetracycline-sensitive genital *Mycoplasmas* were considered a possible explanation of these findings. Some studies have found an apparent connection between cervical colonization with *Ureaplasma urealyticum* or *Mycoplasma hominis* and prematurity. Kundsin isolated *Mycoplasma* more commonly from placentae after perinatal loss than after normal outcomes.[27] However, recent prospective studies have not been able to confirm the association with prematurity.[23] *Chlamydia* is associated with abortion in cattle, and recently Martin and colleagues reported that cervical colonization with *Chlamydia* at 19 weeks was associated with a 10-fold risk for fetal or neonatal death from premature labor, premature rupture of membranes, or chorioamnionitis.[28]

A study of pregnant women in a Guatemalan Indian village documented a high rate of upper respiratory infections, diarrheal illnesses, urinary tract infections, vaginitis, and silent infections with enteric pathogens such as *Shigella, Entamoeba histolytica,* and enteroviruses. Eleven percent of those tested showed seroconversion during pregnancy to cytomegalovirus or herpes virus.[29] Forty-two percent of the newborns had elevated cord blood levels of IgM, reflecting a very high rate of exposure to intrauterine infection. Although in this small sample, birth weight was not correlated with presence of elevated cord serum IgM, the rate of low birth weight in the village is extraordinarily high, and the authors propose that repeated infections of the pregnant woman can impair the woman's nutritional status and indirectly reduce fetal growth.

Maternal Cigarette Smoking

Smoking is strongly associated with low birth weight, prematurity, intrauterine growth retardation, fetal death in utero, neonatal death, placenta previa, placental abruption, and premature rupture of the fetal membranes.[30] Perinatal mortality among smokers is increased because of fetal deaths from anoxia and of neonatal deaths because of premature delivery. Various mechanisms have been proposed. Nicotine crosses the placenta and carbon monoxide in the smoke results in production of maternal and fetal carboxyhemoglobin which reduces the oxygen-carrying capacity of both maternal and fetal blood.

Lack of Prenatal Care

Even though little is done in conventional prenatal care that might influence either birth weight or length of gestation, prenatal care always predicts a better outcome. In the multivariate analysis of Eisner et al, lack of prenatal care was the single most important factor associated with low birth weight in the United States.[31]

Iatrogenic Prematurity

Failure to establish gestational age prior to elective repeat cesarean birth has led to iatrogenic prematurity. This can be totally prevented by routine use of ultrasound in mid-pregnancy to confirm gestational age[32] or by the simpler expedient of allowing spontaneous labor to begin before a cesarean is repeated and by encouraging vaginal birth after previous cesarean.

Induced Abortion and Premature Birth

Older papers from Eastern Europe alleged prematurity as a frequent complication of induced abortion. A review of recent studies of the problem concludes that there is no measurable risk for later pregnancy from legal abortion as currently practiced.[33] Many had been concerned that, while one induced abortion might be safe, multiple abortions could still confer risk. In a large Boston study, it initially appeared that women reporting two or more prior induced abortions did suffer a number of reproductive complications in the next pregnancy. However, appropriate statistical control with multiple regression analysis found multiple induced abortions to be associated only with first trimester bleeding, abnormal presentations, and rupture of the membranes before onset of labor, but not with low birth weight, prematurity, or perinatal loss.[34]

Previous Spontaneous Loss

In contrast to the case of induced abortion, previous spontaneous abortion or later reproductive loss is highly correlated with subsequent prematurity and low birth weight.[35] The study of Bakketeig et al in Norway found that women whose first-born infant was low birth weight and preterm had a 6- to 12-fold increased risk of giving birth to a second infant preterm and low birth weight by comparison to the total population of mothers having two births during the same time period.[36]

Sexual Intercourse during Pregnancy

That sexual relations might endanger pregnancy has been considered since ancient times. The literature affords considerable evidence for direct effects of intercourse and of orgasm upon the pregnancy, as for example, documented uterine contractions and slowing of the fetal heart rate.[37] In several studies, Naeye and colleagues have related intercourse in late pregnancy to amniotic infection syndrome and premature birth.[38] In reporting a prospective study from Denmark, Andersen and Fuchs note that the frequency of sexual activity declines as pregnancy advances, so that women questioned early in the third trimester are much more likely to report recent intercourse than those questioned at term and that a causal relationship between intercourse and prematurity is not yet proven.[39]

Illegitimacy

Illegitimacy is consistently associated with low birth weight.[31] A marriage license cannot change the rate of intrauterine fetal growth, but being unmarried undoubtedly serves to identify individuals with fewer social supports and probably at greater risk for nutritional deprivation as well.

Interaction of Multiple Factors

Miller and Merritt reported a careful study of infant size as it related to a number of maternal factors in a US data set.[40] Among white, singleton births to women with no maternal illness, they found that seven "behavioral characteristics" accounted for most of the observed differences in incidence of low birth weight: low maternal weight for height, low maternal weight gain in pregnancy, lack of prenatal care, delivery before the mother's 17th birthday or after her 35th, cigarette smoking, and the use of addicting drugs or alcohol (Table 3-4). If none of the factors were present, the incidence of LBW was only 1%. Among nonwhites, the incidence of LBW was 6.2% when none of the factors was present.[40]

High rates of LBW are found in populations where many factors operate at once. Eisner and colleagues used a multivariate analysis to study all singleton liveborns in the United States in 1974. These factors were important: nonwhite race, previous reproductive loss, short interpregnancy interval, out of wedlock birth, lack of prenatal care, maternal age under 18 or over 35 years.[31]

Table 3-4
Incidence of Low Birth Weight According to Number of Behavioral Conditions* Present among White Mothers†

No. of variables present per pregnancy	Mothers	LBW infants *Number*	LBW infants *Percent*
0	624	6	1.0
1	506	34	6.7
2	168	17	10.1
>3	45	13	28.9

*As defined in the text.
†Source: Miller and Merritt, p 28,[40] by permission.

Maternal Stress and Prematurity

In their discussion of the many personal and social factors that can affect birth weight and gestation age, Bragonier and colleagues propose that such things as nutritional deprivation, smoking and substance abuse, maternal work, short interpregnancy intervals, poor hygiene, coitus, and colonization with bacteria, magnified by an inadequate system of social supports, in an individual already at risk because of age, or small body, all potentiate each other leading to a generalized stress reaction which then precipitates premature delivery.[41]

CAUSES OF SHORT GESTATION

Most of the factors associated with LBW are also associated with short gestation. Fedrick and Anderson[7] defined "premature" as born after spontaneous labor prior to 37 weeks and with birth weight less than 2500 g. Associated factors were: young maternal age, low socioeconomic class, low maternal weight (less than 50 kg), cigarette smoking, maternal employment for primigravidae but not for multigravidae, past history of pregnancy loss, previous low-birth-weight infant, previous antepartum hemorrhage, bleeding in the present pregnancy, and certain medical illnesses (nephrectomy, hepatitis, and fever during labor associated with ruptured membranes).[7] In the same study, maternal height was not important when weight was controlled, and parity was not important. The effect of prenatal care could not be studied as only six women had received no care.

The Fedrick studies and most others are cross-sectional, that is, they compare all births, or all first births, all second births, etc. An important exception is the work of Bakketeig and colleagues. Using record linkage data from Norway, they identified a large cohort of women who had from one to three births during 1967–1976.[13] They were able to compare first, second, and third births to individual mothers. In summary, their observations were as follows:

Premature births repeat First births had the highest prematurity rate and then the rates declined. An important exception were mothers whose first birth occurred before age 20. For them, prematurity increased with birth order. This is the same observation Puffer and Serrano made earlier in Latin America.[16] The highest risk group were mothers under age 20. First births to women over 35 were also at increased risk for prematurity. Other associations were: illegitimacy, lower educational attainment by the mother or father, bleeding during the pregnancy, position anomalies (breech), congenital anomalies, and of course, low birth weight.

CLINICAL CONTEXTS OF PREMATURE BIRTH

Just as preterm birth and low birth weight are separate but related problems, preterm birth occurs in different clinical contexts. Interventions to prevent premature birth or to improve the outcome must be specific to the clinical context. In a pioneering work, Zlatnick estimated that only 20% or

Table 3-5
Proportion of Admissions and of Deliveries of Preterm Infants by Clinical Context*

Clinical context	Percent of mothers at risk for premature delivery presenting in this fashion	Percent of premature infants that presented in this fashion
In labor, membranes intact		
1A Cervix < 3 cm	20.9	11.6
1B Cervix 3–4 cm	2.9	3.5
2 Cervix > 5 cm	9.7	12.8
Premature rupture of fetal membranes		
3 Not in labor	18.9	21.5
4 In labor	16.5	19.2
Other		
5 Bleeding	13.6	11.0
6 Maternal/fetal illness	14.6	16.3
7 Fetal death in utero	2.9	4.1
	N = 206 mothers	N = 172 infants

*Source: Stubblefield,[43] by permission.

so of premature births might be prevented by drugs that stop uterine contractions, because the balance of the patients present to the hospital with fetal membranes already ruptured, or in preterm labor too far advanced to be stopped.[42] We expanded on his work and reviewed all cases of women presenting at risk for premature delivery to Boston Hospital for Women during a four-month period April 1, 1977, through July 31, 1977.[43] Based on the problems presented to the clinician, we could identify six different clinical contexts (Table 3-5). Those in early preterm labor with fetal membranes intact made up 20.9% of the admissions at risk for preterm delivery, but contributed only 10% of the preterm births because half the time labor stopped spontaneously or was stopped by treatment with medication. Those in more advanced preterm labor made up a smaller portion of the sample, but usually went on to preterm delivery. The most important groups were those with fetal membranes already ruptured at time of admission, totaling 35.6% of admissions at risk, and contributing 40% of the preterm births. Infant outcomes are shown in Table 3-6. Those presenting in early premature labor contributed relatively few perinatal deaths. Advanced premature labor and premature rupture of the membranes contributed the most to perinatal wastage.

EPIDEMIOLOGY OF PREMATURE RUPTURE OF MEMBRANES

Studies of prematurity for the most part, have made no attempt to determine the epidemiology of these specific clinical problems, but have looked only at overall indicators of prematurity, usually births prior to 37 weeks, or low birth weight. A notable exception is the work of Naeye. He studied 5230 women each of whom contributed two successive births to the collaborative perinatal study.[44] Preterm rupture of the fetal membranes was defined as rupture of the membranes occurring before the onset of labor and prior to 259 days from start of the last menses. Preterm rupture of the membranes was associated with coitus in conjunction with the pathological finding of chorioamnionitis and was seen when surgery or instrumentation of the cervix had occurred. There was a strong tendency to repeat, with 21% of second pregnancies exhibiting preterm premature rupture of the membranes if that had happened in the first pregnancy. As reviewed by Kitzmiller, there is considerable evidence for an association between bacterial amnionitis and preterm premature rupture of the membranes.[45] The difficulty has been in determining which came first, the infection weakening the membranes and allowing rupture or a secondary infection occurring after rupture.

Table 3-6
Infant Outcomes by Clinical Context at Time of Admission to Hospital: Percent Premature Perinatal Deaths, Rate of Malformation, and Rate of Respiratory Distress Syndrome (RDS)

Clinical context*	Number of		Prematurity (%)	Perinatal death (%)	Malformation (%)	RDS (%)
	Mothers	*Infants*				
1A	43	44	45.5	6.8	2.3	9.1
1B	6	7	85.7	28.6	0	0
2	20	22	100.0	40.9	4.5	13.6
3	39	39	94.9	23.1	5.1	35.9
4	34	35	94.3	14.3	2.9	20.0
5	28	28	67.9	14.3	7.1	17.9
6	30	31	90.3	19.4	9.7	19.4
7	6	7	100.0	100.0	14.3	NA
Totals	206	213	80.7	21.1	5.2	18.3

*As defined in Table 3-5.

STRATEGIES FOR PREVENTION OF PREMATURITY AND LOW BIRTH WEIGHT

Rheumatic heart disease can be reduced by primary measures, such as reducing crowding, and improving living conditions so that fewer will develop strep pharyngitis, and by secondary prevention, treating cases of strep pharyngitis with penicillin before postinfectious complications can develop. Similarly, premature birth could be prevented primarily and secondarily. Primary prevention would include such measures as improved living conditions, encouraging marriage to maximize social support, delaying childbearing until adolescence is completed, spacing births, providing good nutrition during childhood so that future mothers attain their genetic potential size, providing good nutrition during pregnancy, avoiding sexual contact with infected partners, avoiding cigarette smoking, and providing prenatal care. Secondary measures would include teaching women and their obstetric providers to recognize premature labor early when it can be successfully treated with drugs that stop uterine contractions. Furthermore, the morbidity and mortality after premature birth can be dramatically reduced by expert medical care, most especially by community-wide programs that transfer high-risk women to tertiary care centers prior to birth.[46]

Tocolytic Therapy

A variety of drugs have been used to stop the contracting uterus (tocolysis). In the United States, intravenous ethanol and, more recently, $beta_2$ agonists such as ritodrine and terbutaline are employed.[47] Newer agents such as the calcium channel blockers will be used in the future. Ethanol is more effective than placebo,[48] and $beta_2$ agonists are more effective than ethanol.[47] However, none of the present agents are of much benefit in prolonging pregnancy if the uterine cervix has dilated to more than 4 cm when treatment starts or if the fetal membranes have ruptured. Herron and colleagues demonstrated, in a pilot study, that preterm deliveries were reduced in a high-risk group by intensive education of patients and medical staff to early signs of premature labor so that tocolytic medications could be used before it was too late.[49] These findings are hopeful. However, our analysis of the clinical contexts of preterm birth in the United States suggests that even if we had drugs that were 100% effective for early preterm labor, such regimens would make only a small, albeit important, contribution to the problem of preventing premature birth. We will have to provide more primary prevention.

RECENT REDUCTIONS IN U.S. NEONATAL MORTALITY

Analysis of national data by Lee et al suggests there has been no national decrease in the proportion of infants that are LBW over a 25-year interval ending in 1975.[50] Thus the marked improvement in survival was achieved by better care of the small infant. Subsequently, a different point of view was expressed by David and Siegel from their analysis of North Carolina data.[51] They found a reduction in the proportion of LBW babies born from 1968–1975 ("better babies") and calculate that this accounted for 34% of the fall in neonatal mortality that occurred in North Carolina during that time period. The remaining proportion of the improvement is attributed to better care. Kessel and colleagues, analyzing US statistics from 1970 to 1980, demonstrated a significant decline in the incidence of low birth weight over that period.[52] Of interest, the major portion of the reduction in low birth weight was in reduced births of term low-birth-weight infants. There was only a modest decrease in preterm low birth weight.

When viewed over the entire period from 1950, we can see that although there has indeed been a decrease in proportion of low-birth-weight deliveries in the United States, the

Table 3-7
Rates* of Low Birth Weight in the United States from 1950 to 1980†

Year	Births		Total population
	White	*Nonwhite*	
1950	70.0	100.0	78.0
1970	64.4	129.7	73.9
1975	58.5	121.7	68.4
1980	53.2	117.0	63.1

*Rates are per 1000.
†Sources: Lee et al[50] and Kessel et al.[52]

decrease is not great and most of the decrease occurred because of improvement in low birth weight in the majority, white population. The rate of low birth weight was lower for blacks in 1950 than in 1980, and although this has been attributed to poor reporting of black births during the early years of the period, it is clear that the decrease in low birth weight for the nonwhite population has been slight (Table 3-7). To a very great extent, prematurity and low birth weight are "social diseases." In every society where low birth weight and infant mortality have been studied, the higher income groups always enjoy much lower rates of prematurity and low birth weight than the poor. In countries with very high rates of infant mortality, the upper classes have infant mortality rates as low as any in the world.[53] If we wish to have a rate of prematurity as low as Sweden's, we may have to reform our society in a way that approaches Sweden's, where all are assured a minimum adequate standard of living.

REFERENCES

1. World Health Organization: The incidence of low birth weight: A critical review of available information. *World Health Statistics Q* 1980;33:197–224.
2. Sabbagha RE, Tamura RK, Dal Compl S: *Semin Roentgenol* 1982; 16:190–197.

3. Brenner WE, Edelman DA, Hendricks CH: A standard of fetal growth for the United States of America. *Am J Obstet Gynecol* 1976;126:555–564.
4. Yerushalmy J: Relation of birth weight, gestational age and the rate of intrauterine growth to perinatal mortality. *Clin Obstet Gynecol* 1970;13:107–129.
5. Hoffman HJ, Lundin FE, Bakketeig LS, et al: Classification of births by weight and gestational age for future studies of prematurity, in Reed DM, Stanley FJ (eds): *The Epidemiology of Prematurity*. Baltimore, Munich, Urban and Schwarzenberg, 1977, pp 297–325.
6. Villar J, Belizan JM: The relative contribution of prematurity and fetal growth retardation to low birth weight in developing and developed societies. *Am J Obstet Gynecol* 1982;143:793–798.
7. Fedrick J, Anderson ABM: Factors associated with spontaneous preterm birth. *Br J Obstet Gynecol* 1976;183:342–350.
8. Guyer B, Wallach LA, Rosen SL: Birth weight standardized neonatal mortality rates and the prevention of low birth weight: How does Massachusetts compare with Sweden? *N Engl J Med* 1982;306:1230–1233.
9. Cawley RH, McKeown T, Record RG: Parental stature and birth-weight. *Am J Hum Genet* 1954;6:448–456.
10. Hardy JB, Mellits ED: Relationship of low birth weight to maternal characteristics of age, parity, education and body size, in Reed DM, Stanley FJ (eds): *The Epidemiology of Prematurity*. Baltimore and Munich, Urban and Schwarzenberg, 1977, pp 105–118.
11. Mata LJ, Urrutia JJ, Kronmal RA, et al: Survival and physical growth in infancy and early childhood: Study of birth weight and gestational age in a Guatemalan Indian Village. *Am J Dis Child* 1975;129:561–566.
12. Susser M, Stein Z: Prenatal nutrition and subsequent development, in Reed DM, Stanley FJ (eds): *The Epidemiology of Prematurity*. Baltimore and Munich, Urban and Schwarzenberg, 1977, pp 177–192.
13. Bakketeig LS, Hoffman HJ: Epidemiology of preterm birth: Results from a longitudinal study of births in Norway, in Elder MG, Hendricks CH (eds): *Preterm Labor*. London, Butterworths, 1981, pp 17–46.
14. Garn SM, Shaw HA, McCabe KD: Effects of socioeconomic status and race on weight-defined and gestational prematurity in the United States, in Reed DM, Stanley FJ (eds): *The Epidemiology of Prematurity*. Baltimore and Munich, Urban and Schwarzenberg, 1977, pp 127–143.

15. Zlatnick FJ, Burmeister LF: Low gynecologic age: An obstetric risk factor. *Am J Obstet Gynecol* 1977;128:183–186.
16. Puffer RR, Serrano CV: Birth weight, maternal age, and birth order: Three important determinants in infant mortality. *Pan Am Health Organization Scientific Publication* 1975;294:15.
17. Winikoff B: The effects of birth spacing on child and maternal health. *Stud Fam Plann* 1983;14:231–245.
18. Fedrick J, Adelstein P: Influence of pregnancy spacing on outcome of pregnancy. *Br Med J* 1973;4:753–756.
19. Meyer MB: Effects of maternal smoking and altitude on birth weight and gestation, in Reed DM, Stanley FJ (eds): *The Epidemiology of Prematurity.* Baltimore and Munich, Urban and Schwarzenberg, 1977, pp 81–101.
20. Niswander KR: Obstetric factors related to prematurity, in Reed DM, Stanley FJ (eds): *The Epidemiology of Prematurity.* Baltimore and Munich, Urban and Schwarzenberg, 1977, pp 249–268.
21. Friedman E, Neff R: *Pregnancy Hypertension: A Systematic Evaluation of Clinical Diagnostic Criteria.* Acton, MA, Publishing Sciences Group, 1977.
22. Charles D, Hurry DJ: Cervical incompetence, in Fuchs F, Stubblefield PG (eds): *Preterm Birth: Causes, Prevention, and Management.* New York, Macmillan Inc, 1984, pp 98–111.
23. Polk BF: Infectious processes and preterm labor, in Fuchs F, Stubblefield PG (eds): *Preterm Birth: Causes, Prevention, and Management.* New York, Macmillan Inc, 1984, pp 86–97.
24. Driscoll SG, cited in Reid DE, Ryan KR, Benirschke K (ed): *Principles and Management of Human Reproduction.* Philadelphia, WB Saunders, 1972, p 756.
25. Naeye RL, Peters EC: Amniotic fluid infection with intact membranes leading to perinatal death: A prospective study. *Pediatrics* 1978;61:171–177.
26. Elder HA, Santamarina BAG, Smith S, et al: The natural history of asymptomatic bacteriuria in the clinical course and the outcome of pregnancy. *Am J Obstet Gynecol* 1971;111:441.
27. Kundsin RB, Driscoll SG, Pelletier PA: Ureaplasma urealyticum incriminated in perinatal morbidity and mortality. *Science* 1981; 213:474–476.
28. Martin DH, Koutsky L, Eschenbach DA, et al: Prematurity and perinatal mortality in pregnancies complicated by maternal chlamydia trachomatis infection. *JAMA* 1982;1247:1585–1588.
29. Urritia JJ, Mata LJ, Trent F, et al: Infection and low birth weight in a developing country. *Am J Dis Child* 1975;129:558–561.

30. Meyer MB, Tonascia JA: Maternal smoking, pregnancy complications, and perinatal mortality. *Am J Obstet Gynecol* 1977;128: 494–502.
31. Eisner V, Brazie JV, Pratt MW, et al: The risk of low birthweight. *Am J Public Health* 1979;69:887–893.
32. Frigoletto FD, Phillippe M, Davies IJ, et al: Avoiding iatrogenic prematurity with elective repeat cesaerean section without the routine use of amniocentesis. *Am J Obstet Gynecol* 1980;137: 521–524.
33. Hogue CJR, Cates W, Tietze C: The effects of induced abortion on subsequent reproduction. *Epidemiol Rev* 1982;4:66–94.
34. Linn S, Schoenbaum SC, Monson RR, et al: The relationship between induced abortion and outcome of subsequent pregnancies. *Am J Obstet Gynecol* 1983;146:136–140.
35. Schoenbaum SC, Monson RR, Stubblefield PG, et al: Outcome of the delivery following an induced or spontaneous abortion. *Am J Obstet Gynecol* 1980;136:19–24.
36. Bakketeig LS, Hoffman HJ, Harley EE: The tendency to repeat gestational age and birth weight in successive births. *Am J Obstet Gynecol* 1979;135:1086–1102.
37. Goodlin RC, Schmidt W, Creevy DC: Uterine tension and fetal heart rate during maternal orgasm. *Obstet Gynecol* 1972;39: 125–127.
38. Naeye RL, Ross S: Coitus and chorioamnionitis: A prospective study. *Early Hum Dev* 1982;6:91–97.
39. Anderson LR, Fuchs F: Sexual activity and preterm birth, in Fuchs F, Stubblefield PG (eds): *Preterm Birth: Causes, Prevention, and Management.* New York, Macmillan Inc, 1984, pp 112–120.
40. Miller HC, Merritt TA: *Fetal Growth in Humans.* Chicago, London, Yearbook Medical publishers, 1977.
41. Bragonier JR, Cushner IM, Hobel CJ: Social and personal factors in the etiology of preterm birth, in Fuchs F, Stubblefield PG (eds): *Preterm Birth: Causes, Prevention, and Management.* New York, Macmillan Inc, 1984, pp 64–87.
42. Zlatnick FJ: The applicability of labor inhibition to the problem of prematurity. *Am J Obstet Gynecol* 1972;113:704–706.
43. Stubblefield PG: Causes and prevention of preterm birth: An overview, in Fuchs F, Stubblefield PG (eds): *Preterm Birth: Causes, Prevention, and Management.* New York, Macmillan Inc, 1984, pp 15–17.
44. Naeye RL: Factors that predispose to premature rupture of the fetal membranes. *Obstet Gynecol* 1982;60:93–98.

45. Kitzmiller JL: Preterm premature rupture of the membranes, in Fuchs F, Stubblefield PG (eds): *Preterm Birth: Causes, Prevention, and Management.* New York, Macmillan Inc, 1984, pp 298–322.
46. Scott KE, Peddle LJ, Rees EP: Impact of regional organization and planned services to reduce perinatal mortality, in Fuchs F, Stubblefield PG (eds): *Preterm Birth: Causes, Prevention, and Management.* New York, Macmillan Inc, 1984, pp 348–376.
47. Creasy RK, Katz M: Basic research and clinical experience with B-adrenergic tocolytics in the United States, in Fuchs F, Stubblefield PG (eds): *Preterm Birth: Causes, Prevention, and Management.* New York, Macmillan Inc, 1984, pp 150–170.
48. Fuchs F, Fuchs AR: Ethanol for the prevention of preterm birth, in Fuchs F, Stubblefield PG (eds): *Preterm Birth: Causes, Prevention, and Management.* New York, Macmillan Inc, 1984, pp 207–222.
49. Herron MA, Katz M, Creasy RK: Evaluation of a preterm birth prevention program: Preliminary report. *Obstet Gynecol* 1982; 59:452–456.
50. Lee K, Paneth N, Gartner LM, et al: Neonatal mortality: An analysis of the recent improvement in the United States. *Am J Public Health* 1980;70:15–21.
51. David RJ, Siegel E: Decline in neonatal mortality 1968–1977: Better babies or better care? *Pediatrics* 1983;71:531–540.
52. Kessel SS, Villar J, Herendes HW, et al: The changing pattern of low birth weight in the United States: 1970–1980. *JAMA* 1984; 251:1978–1982.
53. Wray JB: *Child Health in the Third World.* Paper presented at the University of Connecticut Symposium on International Health, Farmington, Conn, May 20, 1983.

CHAPTER 4

ELECTRONIC FETAL MONITORING

Henry Klapholz, MD
Susan Bassett, MD

INTRODUCTION

In 1980, there were 3,612,000 children born alive in the United States. That year, 63,210 (17.5/1000) suffered perinatal demises.[1] Of those children who survived, 11,000–14,000 (3–4/1000) school-aged children will be diagnosed as severely mentally retarded, and 7000–9000 (2–2.5/1000) will be physically handicapped by cerebral palsy.[2] Some of those deaths and handicaps are not preventable because they are due to causes beyond the control of the obstetrician, but it is estimated that 10% of mental retardation,[3] 40% of cerebral palsy,[4] and 30% of perinatal mortality[5] is attributable to peripartum events. The goal of fetal surveillance is to identify the fetus at risk and appropriately intervene to prevent anoxic damage.

Auscultation of the fetal heart tones for the detection of fetal distress has been practiced for over 160 years. It was not until the 1950s that continuous monitoring of the fetus during labor by electronic means was proposed as a way to prevent poor fetal outcome.[6] Today, 90% of patients at some centers are monitored continuously during labor;[7] however, there is evidence that techniques now available for fetal monitoring have limited success in accurately predicting fetal outcome. This chapter will review the pathophysiology of fetal asphyxia and the ability of fetal monitoring to predict its occurrence and consequences.

EFFECTS OF FETAL ASPHYXIA

There is strong evidence that severe peripartum asphyxia can cause fetal death and neurological impairment. The evidence comes from both animal experimentation and clinical studies. Myers[8] showed that within 10 min of total asphyxia, fetal monkeys suffered brain damage, and that after 25 min, they died. Anoxic damage that was severe enough to cause brain damage usually resulted in myocardial ischemia which contributed to death. Autopsies showed damage primarily to the brain stem areas. These areas are rarely affected in asphyxiated neonates, but total asphyxia is a rare event except under experimental conditions.

Partial asphyxia in monkeys causes a different pattern of brain damage. Myers et al[9] created prolonged partial asphyxia by hyperstimulating the maternal uterus of monkeys with oxytocin, and found cerebral swelling, flattening of convolutions, and cerebral herniation. He also found status marmoratus, and cortical atrophy in a 6-month-old monkey who exhibited motor deficits after prolonged partial asphyxia.[10] These changes were similar to those seen in human infants who had died after birth asphyxia or perinatal trauma.[11] Infants whose anoxic insult was severe enough to cause brain damage usually manifested impaired neurological function prior to death.

The consequences of severe perinatal anoxia in humans include fetal or neonatal death, and mental or neurological damage. Perinatal mortality is often secondary to multiple causes (Table 4-1), prematurity being a leading risk factor. It is often difficult to separate out the role of asphyxia; however, MacDonald et al[12] showed that neonatal asphyxia increased

Table 4-1
Causes of Perinatal Mortality

	Percent
Intrapartum	
Cord and placental complications	29.9
Antepartum	
Placental infarction	24.4
Congenital malformation	21.0
Toxemia	9.6

the risk of death at all gestational ages and weights. Between 1970 and 1975, 9% of preterm infants, and 0.5% of term infants died secondary to asphyxia at Magee-Women's Hospital.

Scott[13] followed children who had had an Apgar score of zero at one minute (15 infants) or who had failed to establish spontaneous respiration by 20 min (33 infants). There was a 52% mortality rate, with 13 of the deaths presumed secondary to asphyxia. Twenty of the 23 survivors had some neurological problem, although most abnormalities disappeared by 6 weeks. Seventeen of the 23 survivors were normal in long-term follow-up, six had cerebral palsy, and two of those with spastic quadraplegia were also severely mentally retarded. Brown[14] followed 14,020 children born in Edinburgh in 1974: 5.4% were severely asphyxiated as evidenced by the fact that 88% required endotracheal intubation, 80% had Apgars of less than 3 at 5 min, and 63% had abnormal acid–base studies. Eleven percent of the asphyxiated babies (0.59% of the total) had abnormal neurological examinations in the nursery, and 20% of those (0.12% of the total) went on to develop cerebral palsy. He notes, "asphyxia occurs in 54 per 1000 liveborn infants, of whom only seven are likely to be at risk of permanent brain damage."

Estimates of significant neurological handicap attributable to asphyxia vary from 6%[15] to 22%.[16] Unfortunately, many of the early studies do not consider potential confounding variables such as gestational age, growth retardation, birth methods, or the presence of birth trauma.

In 1980, Mulligan et al[17] showed that survival following asphyxia increased with gestational age and that the incidence of severe impairment decreased with gestational age. In their study, severely asphyxiated infants of over 36 weeks of gestation had a 19% incidence of severe sequelae, as opposed to a 25% incidence in those infants of less than 30 weeks' gestation. Nelson and Ellenberg[18] stated that infants weighing 1500–2500 g had a three to four times higher incidence of neurological impairment than infants over 2500 g. Perinatal asphyxia has been correlated with an increased incidence of intraventricular hemorrhage in the preterm infant.[19] Despite the increased risk of cerebral palsy with prematurity, the majority of infants with cerebral palsy are delivered at term because the volume of term deliveries is so much higher.

Intrauterine growth retardation and states of chronic anoxia may also predispose to neurological damage. In an epidemiologic study of cerebral palsy, Dale and Stanley[20] showed that 17.8% of cerebral palsy infants as opposed to 2.9% of controls were intrauterine growth-retarded. Nelson and Browman did not confirm the association of intrauterine growth retardation and cerebral palsy.[21] Infants who show neurological abnormalities during the newborn period, such as seizures, hypertonia, hypotonia, or feeding problems, have a higher incidence of later developing cerebral palsy.

The correlation between birth asphyxia and mental retardation is less clear. Many cases of severe mental retardation are due to chromosomal abnormalities. Stein and Susser[22] noted that over 90% of significant mental retardation is attributable to antenatal events beyond the scope of present-day detection techniques. Only 1–2% of mental retardation is thought to be secondary to asphyxia. There is considerable overlap between mental retardation and cerebral palsy. Fifty percent of children with cerebral palsy will be expected to have normal IQ scores, but 25% of them will be severely retarded.[18] Ten to 20% of children with severe mental retardation will have cerebral palsy.[18] In a study by Thomson et al,[15] the mean IQ of a group of asphyxiated children was the same as controls; however, two of the 29 infants who had suffered asphyxia had both cerebral palsy and severe mental retardation.

In summary, perinatal asphyxia can lead to death, cerebral palsy, or mental retardation. Fortunately, the majority of asphyxiated infants, especially those at term, will escape permanent damage and will be normal in long-term follow-up. The goal of fetal heart rate monitoring is to detect fetal hypoxia before it causes irreparable damage.

FETAL HEART RATE MONITORING

The earliest reference to fetal heart rate auscultation was in 1650 by Marsac, but it was not until 1822 that auscultation was used to detect fetal distress.[6] In 1893, Von Winckel proposed that a fetal heart rate in the range of 120–160 beats/min was associated with nonasphyxiated babies. Rates outside of this range were frequently associated with compromised neonates. Bradycardias were traditionally grounds for immediate intervention, especially if they occurred in the presence of meconium. The frequently inconsistent and often contradictory results obtained by this approach caused many to question its validity.

In 1968, Benson and coworkers[23] concluded that there is no single auscultatory finding that predicts fetal distress. This apparent insensitivity of auscultation is explained by three factors: (1) intermittent heart rate sampling consitutes less than 2% of the time a mother spends in labor;[6] (2) fetal heart rates often cannot be heard by auscultation during a uterine contraction; and (3) auscultation is often unable to detect subtle or brief changes in heart rate.

Haverkamp et al[24] and Kelso et al[25] proposed that it is acceptable to monitor high- and low-risk patients by auscultation. Their sample sizes may have been too small to prove the premise that auscultation is as sensitive as fetal heart rate monitoring to detect fetal compromise, as the endpoints of perinatal mortality and neurological impairment occur so infrequently.

In the 1950s, Hon[26] and Caldeyro-Barcia and Alvares[27] established the principles of electronic fetal heart rate monitoring in simultaneous research efforts in the United States and Uruguay. For the first time, fetal heart tones could be recorded throughout labor, and specific changes in heart rate related to contractions could be noted.

Techniques for fetal heart rate monitoring have changed over the years. The first electrically measured and recorded fetal electrocardiogram was in 1906.[28] The major problem associated with abdominal wall fetal electrocardiography is the presence of a large maternal signal that makes detection of low-amplitude fetal signals difficult. Maternal muscular electrical artifact also diminishes the value of this technique by creating false trigger signals that are counted as fetal heartbeats. In selected thin individuals, the technique may be employed today, and can supply valuable information if the fetal heart rate is rapid and the maternal one is slow.

A more useful technique is the Doppler ultrasound method. This relies upon a beam of ultrasound, usually at 2.5 MHz, that strikes the moving fetal heart and is reflected back at a frequency that has been altered by the velocity of the reflective surfaces. The magnitude and frequency of the Doppler shift so produced is a function of the heart wall, valvular, and blood movement, and thus can be used to time cardiac events. The major limitation of this technique is that the precision of timing is obscured somewhat due to uncertainty in the exact timing of reflected signals, thus the technology generates more variability in fetal heart than is acutally present. Newer machines that employ autocorrelation to estimate the heart rate still do not have the precision obtained by direct recording via fetal scalp electrode.

All methods of monitoring will give information about the fetal heart rate changes that can then be correlated with changes in uterine activity. There are three classic patterns of fetal heart rate first described by Hon and Caldeyro-Barcia.

Early decelerations are symmetric with respect to contractions, beginning and ending simultaneously with their onset and ending. The depth is proportional to the magnitude of the contraction as well as the length. Late decelerations are symmetric as well but begin 20 or more seconds after the onset of the contraction. The depth of these decelerations is similarly related to the magnitude and duration of uterine activity. Variable decelerations may begin at any time and may have a variable shape. They are, however, generally characterized by sharp rises and falls in rate over short periods of time.

Early decelerations are felt to be innocuous and indicative of fetal head compression. They may be blocked by the administration of atropine to the fetus or mother, indicating a vagally mediated mechanism. Variable decelerations are secondary to umbilical cord compression and are vagally mediated. The fetal baroreceptors sense an increase in peripheral resistance when the umbilical artery pressure increases with the extrinsic compression of the cord. This creates a profound vagal discharge, followed by a prompt bradycardia which recovers after the release of cord occlusion. Variable decelerations do not occur in phase with a contraction. Variable decelerations are not thought to indicate fetal compromise unless they are severe or in an atypical pattern.[29]

Late decelerations are considered evidence of uteroplacental insufficiency and are often associated with poor fetal outcome. The decelerations may be secondary to both an increase in vagal discharge and direct myocardial depression. The drop in fetal heart rate begins after the peak intensity of the uterine contraction and returns to the baseline after the completion of the contraction.

Data from animal studies confirm that fetal asphyxia can lead to fetal heart rate aberrations. Murata et al[30] showed that fetal rhesus monkeys exhibited late decelerations and loss of accelerations during terminal asphyxia. Barcroft created variable decelerations in sheep by clamping the umbilical cord.[31] Other studies confirmed that asphyxia (created by clamping the maternal aorta) and acute hypoxemia (created by altering inspired gas content) can produce changes in fetal heart rate which are similar to those seen in humans.[32,33]

Ominous fetal heart rate patterns during labor are those which exhibit late decelerations and severe or atypical variable decelerations, especially in the absence of variability[34] or accelerations.[35] In human infants, ominous fetal heart rate tracings correlated well with acidosis[36] and were predictive of neonatal neurological abnormalities in both the preterm[37] and term infant. Painter et al[38] showed that 37% of high-risk term infants with ominous fetal heart rate patterns had abnormal neurological examinations at one year of age and that 91% of the abnormal neurological examinations were predicted by abnormal fetal heart rate tracings. Schifrin and Dame[39] found only two depressed babies in 307 normal heart tracings and found that the three intrauterine fetal deaths that occurred subsequent to monitoring all had ominous tracings. Ingemarsson et al[7] considered the impact of fetal monitoring by comparing fetal outcomes from three distinct time periods. There was a significant decrease in infants with low Apgars as the incidence of fetal monitoring increased. For babies with low Apgars that went on to have neurological impairment, 35.2% were born during a time when few patients were monitored versus 4.6% when 90% were monitored.

Randomized trials of electronic fetal monitoring by Haverkamp et al,[24,40] Wood et al,[41] and Kelso et al[25] did not show an immediate benefit from monitoring. In contrast, Renou et al[42] showed a major decrease in neurologic damage in monitored patients. In their 1976 study, high-risk patients

Eastern College of Nursing Library

were randomized to monitored or auscultated groups. There was one stillbirth thought secondary to asphyxia in the auscultated group. Thirteen babies in the auscultated group had neurological abnormalities compared to two in the monitored group, and four of the auscultated infants showed evidence of brain damage on long-term follow-up. Cord pH, P_{CO_2} and P_{O_2} values were better in the monitored group.

Clinical studies reviewing the impact of fetal monitoring on the incidence of cerebral palsy and mental retardation have multiple problems:

1. A prospective, controlled, blinded study to examine the effect of electronic fetal monitoring on the incidence of mental retardation or cerebral palsy would be impossible to perform. Quilligan[43] estimated that it would take a 7- to 10-year follow-up of 1500 live births to verify an effect of electronic fetal monitoring on mental retardation if monitoring halved the incidence. All of the infants in the group would need to be followed to prevent bias.

2. During the time required to detect the effect of electronic fetal monitoring on mental retardation or cerebral palsy, many changes in obstetrical and neonatal practices and techniques will have occurred that directly impact on the incidence and severity of the disorders.

3. There are currently no reliable neonatal evaluations that will predict long-term outcome. Apgar scores do not correlate well with fetal acidosis[38] or the development of cerebral palsy. Seventy-three percent of children with cerebral palsy have a 5-min Apgar score of greater than or equal to 7.[2]

4. Controversy has also arisen about what a "normal" fetal scalp pH should be and what endpoint a particular pH should predict.[46] Severe acidosis can occur with normal fetal heart rate patterns.[38] When electronic fetal monitoring and fetal blood sample pH are used in combination, they have a 7% false-negative rate and an 80% false-positive rate in predicting a 5-min Apgar score of less than 7.[41]

5. The predictive value of electronic fetal monitoring or fetal blood sampling is poor, because the incidence of fetal asphyxia and its consequences is low, especially in a low-risk population.

6. The purpose of fetal surveillance is to intervene before permanent brain damage has occurred. Animal studies show that late decelerations caused by partial asphyxia are present for a long period of time before brain damage occurs.[49] Intervention on the basis of electronic fetal monitoring evident of partial asphyxia is hoped to alter outcome.

There is no precise definition of fetal distress. It is known that hypoxia without acidosis will generally not injure mature neuronal tissues. Elevated tissue lactic acid levels lead to edema and subsequent necrosis with functional loss. This effect is enhanced greatly by the presence of elevated glucose levels and may be diminished by the administration of barbiturate. In order for brain damage to occur, the hypoxic insult needs to be prolonged and severe. This is confirmed by the observation that few hypoxic infants sustain noticeable brain injury.[2] In order to fully appreciate the significance of any study designed to test the hypothesis that electronic fetal monitoring is a reliable predictor of fetal distress, it is appropriate to attempt to define endpoints accurately. Unfortunately, examination of the obstetric literature fails to yield a uniform and agreed upon definition of fetal distress.

Table 4-2 lists various combinations of fetal heart rate patterns that have been associated with adverse outcomes. A recent study,[45] designed to examine the uniformity of expert opinion with regard to the prognostic value of the various abnormal patterns, indicated that considerable discrepancy exists in the obstetrical community. Twelve perinatal physicians, recognized experts in the field of fetal monitoring, were polled in order to determine what course of action they individually would follow if confronted with a patient whose fetus exhibited a given abnormal pattern. Options included observation, delivery, or fetal blood gas sampling. The physicians were first asked to evaluate the degree of fetal compromise that could be associated with a given pattern assuming it was the first abnormal pattern to be encountered in a hypothetical labor. Additionally, it was assumed that each pattern was unequivocally identifiable, that direct fetal monitoring was available to confirm a pattern, that the hypothetical labor was free of other serious predisposing fetal risk factors, and that each pattern appeared in the absence of any other potentially serious abnormal pattern. In addition, it was assumed that a given pattern was repeated and not transient.

The initial impressions of the 14 patterns are shown in Table 4-3. It is evident that the 12 obstetricians differed markedly in the interpretation of four patterns while agreement with respect to five others was nearly perfect. One obstetrician considered none of the patterns as innocuous while another considered only one as ominous. One should note at this time that these obstetricians are all noted teachers who conduct postgraduate courses in fetal monitor techniques and interpretation throughout the country.

The entire group of physicians was then surveyed to determine a suitable course of corrective treatment, if indicated, for each pattern. They were additionally asked to suggest a course of action if in-utero treatment failed. Standard treatment for fetal distress is uniformly accepted to consist of maternal repositioning to the left lateral recumbent position, intravenous fluid administration, and oxygen by mask. Uterotonic agents, if in use, would be discontinued. Table 4-4 shows the variety of responses. It is noted that while overall agreement was 69%, there are some patterns that generated considerable variation in treatment. It is clear that the diversity of interpretation of some patterns may give rise to completely different modalities of therapy that may result in markedly different outcomes. One is hard pressed to attribute good or poor outcome to the technique of fetal monitoring

Table 4-2
Characteristics of 14 Fetal Heart Rate Patterns Presented to Expert Obstetricians for Interpretation

Fetal heart rate pattern*		
Base pattern	*Modifying element(s)*	Other assumptions
1. Late decelerations	Normal baseline variability	
2. Late decelerations	Decreased baseline variability	Variability change not caused by drugs
3. Variable decelerations	Normal baseline variability and normal recovery to the baseline	
4. Variable decelerations	Normal baseline variability and slow recovery to the baseline	
5. Variable decelerations	Decreased baseline variability and normal recovery to the baseline	Variability change not caused by drugs
6. Variable decelerations	Decreased baseline variability and slow recovery to the baseline	Variability change not caused by drugs
7. Marked bradycardia (FHR < 100)	Normal baseline variability	Bradycardia not caused by fetal cardiac arrhythmia or congenital anomaly; variability change not caused by drugs
8. Marked bradycardia (FHR < 100)	Decreased baseline variability	

9. Moderate bradycardia (FHR 100–119)	Normal baseline variability	Bradycardia not caused by fetal cardiac arrhythmia or congenital anomaly; variability change not caused by drugs
10. Moderate bradycardia (FHR 100–119)	Decreased baseline variability	
11. Tachycardia (FHR > 160)	Normal baseline variability	Tachycardia not caused by maternal fever, fetal infection, or drugs; variability change not caused by drugs
12. Tachycardia (FHR > 160)	Decreased baseline variability	
13. Tachycardia (FHR > 160)	Absent baseline variability	
14. Normal baseline rate (FHR 120–160)	Decreased baseline variability	Variability change not caused by drugs

*Recovery time of variable decelerations refers to the interval over which the fetal heart rate (FHR) returns to the normal baseline rate following each deceleration. A lag-time exceeding 15 sec is considered slow recovery.

Table 4-3
Obstetrician Perceptions of Abnormal Fetal Heart Rate Patterns Prior to Corrective Treatment

Fetal heart rate pattern	Number of obstetricians perceiving pattern as		
	Innocuous	*Nonreassuring*	*Ominous*
1. Late decelerations—normal baseline variability	0	9	3
2. Late decelerations—decreased baseline variability	0	5	7
3. Variable decelerations—normal baseline variability, normal recovery	5	7	0
4. Variable decelerations—normal baseline variability, slow recovery	0	10	2
5. Variable decelerations—decreased baseline variability, normal recovery	0	5	7
6. Variable decelerations—decreased baseline variability, slow recovery	0	5	7
7. Marked bradycardia (FHR < 100)—normal baseline variability	0	11	1
8. Marked bradycardia (FHR < 100)—decreased baseline variability	0	5	7
9. Moderate bradycardia (FHR 100–119)—normal baseline variability*	8	2	0

10. Moderate bradycardia (FHR 100–119)—decreased baseline variability*	3	7	0
11. Tachycardia (FHR > 160)—decreased baseline variability	0	12	0
12. Tachycardia (FHR > 160)—decreased baseline variability	0	11	0
13. Tachycardia (FHR > 160)—absent baseline variability	0	1	11
14. Normal baseline rate—decreased baseline variability	0	12	0

*Not asked of all obstetricians.

Table 4-4
Obstetrician Choice of Action Following Corrective Treatment: Two Options Available

Fetal heart rate pattern*	Number choosing to monitor	Number choosing to deliver
1. Late decelerations—normal baseline variability	7	5
2. Late decelerations—decreased baseline variability	2	10
3. Variable decelerations—normal baseline variability, normal recovery	12	0
4. Variable decelerations—normal baseline variability, slow recovery	10	2
5. Variable decelerations—decreased baseline variability, normal recovery	6	6
6. Variable decelerations—decreased baseline variability, slow recovery	3	9
7. Marked bradycardia (FHR < 100)—normal baseline variability	9	3
8. Marked bradycardia (100–119)—decreased baseline variability	2	10
9. Moderate bradycardia (FHR 100–119)—normal baseline variability	10	0
10. Moderate bradycardia (FHR 100–119)—decreased baseline variability†	9	1
11. Tachycardia (FHR > 160)—normal baseline variability‡	11	0
12. Tachycardia (FHR > 160)—decreased baseline variability	8	3
13. Tachycardia (FHR > 160)—absent baseline variability	3	8
14. Normal baseline rate—decreased baseline variability	9	2

*Choice of action is based on continued observation of pattern over several consecutive uterine contractions (approximately 15–30 min) following administration of corrective treatment.
†Not asked of all obstetricians.
‡Obstetrician No. 1 declined to comment on the last four patterns.

itself. Rather, it is not hard to conclude that outcome may well be related to the philosophy of the care-giver.

Carrying this survey one step further, the obstetricians were then asked to indicate their next action if fetal scalp sampling were an available additional diagnostic modality. As Table 4-5 demonstrates, there again was considerable variation in practice, although a large number of physicians chose to utilize fetal pH for confirmation of their initial impression. The reliance on fetal blood sampling to such a large extent seems to confirm the impression that the theoretical construct of monitoring pattern interpretation is an imprecise and somewhat inaccurate one.

The ability of electronic fetal monitoring to alter perinatal mortality is clearer than its effect on long-term neurological outcome. In 1974, Paul and Hon[48] compared a high-risk monitored group of patients to a low-risk unmonitored group of patients and found a perinatal mortality of 1.3/1000 and 4.4/1000, respectively. Perinatal mortality in a group of monitored infants weighing between 1000 and 1500 g was 33% as compared to a 44% mortality rate in the unmonitored group. Tutera and Newman[49] confirmed that high-risk monitored patients had one third the mortality rate of unmonitored low-risk patients admitted in labor. In fact, Wilson and Schifrin[50] ask in an article entitled, "Is Any Pregnancy Low Risk?": "Should we accept perinatal mortality of 5–10/1000 in low-risk patients if we have methods available to lower the rate to 1–2/1000?" Wilson and Schifrin conclude from the above data that all labors should be monitored regardless of risk.

Studies comparing mortality rates in the years before and after fetal monitoring add further evidence revealing a large decrease in perinatal deaths after the introduction of fetal monitoring.[51–53] Mueller-Heubach et al[54] compared statistics from 1970 when no patients were monitored, to 1977 when 72.7% were monitored and found that the intrapartum death rate fell significantly even though there were larger numbers

Table 4-5
Obstetrical Choice of Action Following Corrective Treatment: Three Options Available

	Number choosing to		
Fetal heart rate pattern*	*Monitor*	*Scalp sample*	*Deliver*
1. Late decelerations—normal baseline variability	2	9	1
2. Late decelerations—decreased baseline variability	0	9	3
3. Variability decelerations—normal baseline variability, normal recovery	8	4	0
4. Variable decelerations, normal baseline variability, slow recovery	3	9	0
5. Variable decelerations—decreased baseline variability, normal recovery	2	8	2
6. Variable decelerations—decreased baseline variability, slow recovery	0	8	4
7. Marked bradycardia (FHR < 100) —normal baseline variability	6	6	0
8. Marked bradycardia (FHR < 100) —decreased baseline variability	0	6	6
9. Moderate bradycardia (FHR 100–119)—normal baseline variability†	6	4	0
10. Moderate bradycardia (FHR 100–119)—decreased baseline variability†	0	10	0
11. Tachycardia (FHR > 160)—normal baseline variability	3	8	0
12. Tachycardia (FHR > 160)—decreased baseline variability	1	11	0
13. Tachycardia (FHR > 160)—absent baseline variability	0	9	2
14. Normal baseline rate—decreased baseline variability	3	9	0

*Choice of action is based on continued observation of pattern over several consecutive uterine contractions (approximately 15–30 min) following administration of corrective treatment.
†Not asked of all obstetricians.

of patients in the high-risk category in 1977. Of note, three deaths in the monitored groups occurred in association with unrecognized fetal distress, reinforcing the importance of having qualified personnel review the tracings. Mueller-Heubach et al also found a decrease in the incidence of birth asphyxia in the monitored group.[54] Yeh conducted a retrospective 10-year study of 115,096 births in which 41% were monitored.[55] Perinatal mortality fell as the rate of fetal monitoring increased. Both fetal death and neonatal death rates were significantly lower in the monitored group despite a disproportionately higher number of at-risk pregnancies. The problem with studies using historical controls is that many changes have occurred in obstetrical care over time which would influence outcome.

ANTEPARTUM TESTING

Electronic fetal monitoring can be used to assess fetal well-being prior to the onset of labor. Which test is the most accurate is controversial, but the nonstress test is the quickest and least expensive monitoring modality. Rayburn et al[56] followed 561 high-risk infants and found that those with reactive nonstress tests had a risk of an in-utero death that was less than or equal to that of low-risk patients. There is a 0.3–1% incidence of death within one week of a reactive nonstress test, and a review of those deaths revealed that 53% were secondary to acute changes which could not have been predicted, such an abruption or cord accident.[57] Miyazaki and Miyazaki found that 8% of postterm infants suffered perinatal death or significant fetal distress following a reactive nonstress test. Rh-sensitized, diabetic, and intrauterine-growth-retarded infants[58] have a higher incidence of stillbirth after nonstress testing on a weekly basis, so that additional assessment may be necessary. Schifrin et al[59] followed 131 high-risk patients with contraction stress tests and had no fetal losses within a week of the negative test.

RISKS OF ELECTRONIC FETAL MONITORING

With every technological advance, the risks and benefits must be weighed. Concern has been expressed with regard to the safety of the ultrasound monitors since energy at the 1–10 mW/cm^2 level at the transmitting crystal surface is employed. At this time there are no data to suggest that this level of energy is sufficient to do any harm to the human infant.

There are specific risks from electronic fetal monitoring via the scalp electrode and fetal scalp sampling. The incidence of scalp abscess is 0.3–4.5%; drainage or antibiotic treatment is often required, and osteomyelitis requiring surgical debridement has also been reported.[60] Herpetic infections and gonococcal sepsis[61] have also been reported. Both scalp monitoring and scalp sampling have been associated with cases of significant hemorrhage from scalp lacerations.[62] Maternal risks include lacerations, uterine perforation, increased infection rate, and the discomfort of monitoring itself.[27]

One of the complications of fetal heart rate monitoring is needless intervention in normal, unasphyxiated labors due to physician reaction to a false-positive test. Most studies indicate that the majority of the increase in cesarean section rates is due to a change in the management of cephalopelvic disproportion breeches and preterm infants, rather than intervention because of fetal distress.[63,64] Randomized trials by Kelso et al[25] and Renou et al[42] showed no difference in cesarean section rates in auscultated versus monitored groups, but Haverkamp et al[24,40] showed an increase in the cesarean section rate for fetal distress from 1.2% in auscultated women to 7.4% in monitored women. Fetal blood sampling was able to decrease the cesarean rate for fetal distress to 3%.[40] Monitoring increases the detection of fetal distress and therefore may increase the rate of intervention.

Fetal scalp sampling decreases the rate of false-positive interpretations.

COST

The cost for a cesarean section delivery will be approximately $3000 more than for a vaginal delivery. If only 5% of monitored women are incorrectly diagnosed, an additional $300,000,000 in medical costs will result. The cost of the monitoring must be considered. Currently, the average number of fetal monitors per hospital is three at $8000 per machine, and the average useful life of each of these machines is about five years. Paper, supplies, and maintenance charges average $100 per monitored patient. A total of $200,000,000 in equipment costs will be expended if only 50% of patients are monitored.

CONCLUSIONS

There is considerable evidence that instantaneous fetal heart rate monitoring reflects the state of oxygenation of the fetus. Animal and human data demonstrate a correlation between loss of beat-to-beat variability, the presence of late and variable decelerations, and the loss of reactivity with poor fetal outcome, reduced oxygen saturation levels, and acidosis. Electronic fetal heart rate monitoring is effective in detecting compromised fetuses in high-risk populations in the antepartum and intrapartum period.

Profound asphyxia, sufficient to cause handicapping disorders, is a rare event, and its detection does not ensure the prevention of those handicaps. It is quite possible that abnormal fetal heart rate patterns may simply be markers for events already completed. Since the incidence of intrapartum asphyxia is rare, the predictive value of electronic fetal monitoring will be poor, especially in a low-risk population.

Electronic fetal monitoring is probably one of the causes in the rise in the cesarean section rate. The question that remains to be answered is whether all patients should be subjected to the risks, costs, and discomforts in an attempt to save a few from perinatal morbidity and mortality.

REFERENCES

1. Statistical Abstract of the United States, 1984. US Department of Commerce, Washington, DC.
2. Paneth N, Stark R: Cerebral palsy and mental retardation in relation to indicators of perinatal asphyxia. *Am J Obstet Gynecol* 1983;147:960.
3. Gustavson KH, Hagberg B, Hagberg G, et al: Severe mental retardation in a Swedish country. II Etiologic and pathogenetic aspects of children born 1959–70. *Neuropaediatrie* 1977;8:293.
4. Hagberg B, Hagberg G, Olow I: The changing panorama of cerebral palsy in Sweden 1954–70. II Analysis of the various syndromes. *Acta Paediatr Scand* 1975;69:193.
5. Niswander K: Labor and operative obstetrics, asphyxia in the fetus and cerebral palsy, in Pitkin RM, Zlatnik FJ (eds): *Year Book of Obstetrics and Gynecology.* Chicago, Year Book Medical Publishers, Inc, 1983.
6. Schifrin BS, Suzuki K: Fetal surveillance during labor. *Internat Anesthesiol Clin* 1973;11:17.
7. Ingemarsson E, Ingemarsson I, Svenningsen N: Impact of routine fetal monitoring during labor on fetal outcome with longterm followup. *Am J Obstet Gynecol* 1981;141:29.
8. Myers R: Two patterns of perinatal brain damage and their conditions of occurrence. *Am J Obstet Gynecol* 1972;112:246.
9. Myers R, Beard R, Adamsons K: Brain swelling in the newborn rhesis monkey following prolonged partial asphyxia. *Neurology (NY)* 1969;19:1012.
10. Myer R: Atrophic cortical sclerosis associated with status marmoratus in a perinatally damaged monkey. *Neurology (NY)* 1969; 19:1177.
11. Malamud N: Sequelae of perinatal trauma. *J Neuropathol Exp Neurol* 1959;18:141.
12. MacDonald HM, Mulligan JC, Allen AC, et al: Neonatal asphyxia I: Relationship of obstetric and neonatal complications to neonatal mortality in 38,405 consecutive deliveries. *J Pediatr* 1980;96:898.

13. Scott H: Outcome of very severe birth asphyxia. *Arch Dis Child* 1976;51:712.
14. Brown J, in Hull D (ed): *Recent Advances in Paediatrics.* New York, Churchill Livingstone, 1976, p 35.
15. Thomson A, Searle M, Russell G: Quality of survival after severe birth asphyxia. *Arch Dis Child* 1977;52:620.
16. Brown JK, Purvis RJ, Fofar JO, et al: Neurological aspects of perinatal asphyxia. *Dev Med Child Neurol* 1974;16:567.
17. Mulligan JC, Painter MJ, O'Donoghue PA, et al: Neonatal asphyxia: II Neonatal mortality and long term sequelae. *J Pediatr* 1980;96:903.
18. Nelson KB, Ellenberg JH: Epidemiology of cerebral palsy, in Schoenberg BS (ed): *Advances in Neurology.* New York, Raven Press, 1979, p 19.
19. Flodmark O, Becker L: Correlation between computed tomography and autopsy in premature and fullterm neonates that have suffered perinatal asphyxia. *Radiology* 1980;137:93.
20. Dale A, Stanley F: An epidemiological study of cerebral palsy in Western Australia. *Dev Med Child Neurol* 1980;22:13.
21. Nelson K, Browman S: Perinatal risk factors in children with serious motor and mental handicaps. *Ann Neurol* 1977;2:374.
22. Stein ZA, Susser MW: Mental retardation, in Last JN (ed): *Public Health and Preventive Medicine.* New York, Appleton-Century-Crofts, 1980.
23. Benson R, Shubeck F, Deutschberger J, et al: Fetal heart rate as a predictor of fetal distress. *Obstet Gynecol* 1968;32:259.
24. Haverkamp A, Orleans M, Langendoerfer S: A controlled trial of the differential effects of intrapartum fetal monitoring. *Am J Obstet Gynecol* 1979;134:399.
25. Kelso I, Parsone R, Lawrence D: An assessment of continuous fetal heart rate monitoring in labor: A randomized trial. *Am J Obstet Gynecol* 1978;131:526.
26. Hon EH: Observations on pathologic fetal bradycardia. *Am J Obstet Gynecol* 1959;77:1084.
27. Caldeyro-Barcia R, Alvares H: Proceedings of *Seguendo Congress Latino-American Obstet y Ginecologia.* San Paulo, Brazil, 1954.
28. Banta HD, Thacker S: Assessing the costs and benefits of electronic fetal monitoring. *Obstet Gynecol Surv* 1979;34:627.
29. Krebs HB, Petres RE, Dunn LJ: Intrapartum fetal heart rate monitoring VIII: Atypical variable decelerations. *Am J Obstet Gynecol* 1983;145:297.
30. Murata M, Martin CB, Ikenoue T, et al: Fetal heart rate accelerations and late decelerations during the course of intrauterine

death in chronically catheterized rhesus monkeys. *Am J Obstet Gynecol* 1982;144:218.

31. Barcroft J: *Researches of Prenatal Life.* Springfield, IL, Charles C Thomas, 1947.
32. Ikenoue T, Martin C, Murata Y, et al: Effect of acute hypoxemia and respiratory acidosis on FHR in monkeys. *Am J Obstet Gynecol* 1981;141:797.
33. Boddy K, Dawes GS, Fisher R, et al: Foetal respiratory movements, electrocortical and cardiovascular responses to hypoxaemia and hypercapnia in sheep. *J Physiol* 1974;243:599.
34. Zanini B, Paul R, Huey J: Intrapartum fetal heart rate: Correlation with scalp pH in preterm infant. *Am J Obstet Gynecol* 1980;136:43.
35. Powell OH, Melville A, MacKenna J: Fetal heart rate acceleration in labor: Excellent prognostic indicator. *Am J Obstet Gynecol* 1979;134:36.
36. Sykes G, Johnson P, Ashworth F, et al: Do Apgar scores indicate asphyxia? *Lancet* 1982;1:494.
37. Westgren H, Hormquist P, Ingemarsson I, et al: Intrapartum fetal acidosis in preterm infants: Fetal monitoring and long-term morbidity. *Obstet Gynecol* 1984;63:355.
38. Painter M, Depp R, O'Donoghue P: Fetal heart rate patterns and development in the first year of life. *Am J Obstet Gynecol* 1978;132:271.
39. Schifrin BS, Dame L: Fetal heart rate patterns, Prediction of Apgar score. *JAMA* 1972;219:1322.
40. Haverkamp AD, Thompson H, McFee J, et al: Evaluation of continuous fetal heart rate monitoring in high risk patients. *Am J Obstet Gynecol* 1976;125:310.
41. Wood D, Renou P, Oats J, et al: A controlled trial of fetal heart rate monitoring in a low risk obstetrical population. *Am J Obstet Gynecol* 1981;141:527.
42. Renou P, Chang A, Anderson I, et al: Controlled trial of fetal intensive care. *Am J Obstet Gynecol* 1976;126:470.
43. Quilligan EJ: Summary of fetal monitoring conference. *Int J Gynecol Obstet* 1972;10:163.
44. Cohen AB, Klapholz H, Thompson M: Electronic fetal monitoring in clinical practice. A survey of obstetric opinion. *Med Decision Making* 1982;2:79.
45. Lumley J, McKinnon L, Wood C: Lack of agreement on normal values for fetal scalp blood. *J Obstet Gynecol (Br Commonw)* 1971;8:12.

46. Beard RW, Simons EG: Diagnosis foetal asphyxia in labor. *Br J Anaesth* 1971;43:874.
47. Adamsons K, Myers RE: Late decelerations and brain tolerance of fetal monkey to intrapartum asphyxia. *Am J Obstet Gynecol* 1977;128:893.
48. Paul R, Hon E: Clinical fetal monitoring V: Effect on perinatal outcome. *Am J Obstet Gynecol* 1974;118:529.
49. Tutera G, Newman R: Fetal monitoring: Its effects on perinatal mortality and cesarean section rates and its complications. *Am J Obstet Gynecol* 1975;122:750.
50. Wilson R, Schifrin BS: Is any pregnancy low risk? *Obstet Gynecol* 1980;55:653.
51. Boehm F, Davidson K, Barrett J: The effect of electronic fetal monitoring on the incidence of cesarean section. *Am J Obstet Gynecol* 1981;140:295.
52. Williams R, Chen P: Identifying the sources of the recent decline in perinatal mortality rates in California. *N Engl J Med* 1982;306:207.
53. Neutra R, Fineberg S, Greenland S, et al: The effect of fetal monitoring on neonatal death rates. *N Engl J Med* 1978;299:324.
54. Mueller-Heubach E, MacDonald HM, Joret D, et al: Effects of electronic fetal heart rate monitoring on perinatal outcome and obstetric practices. *Am J Obstet Gynecol* 1980;137:758.
55. Yeh SY, Diaz R, Paul RH: Ten year experience of intrapartum fetal monitoring in Los Angeles County/University of Southern California Medical Center. *Am J Obstet Gynecol* 1982;143:496.
56. Rayburn W, Greene J, Donaldson M: Nonstress testing and perinatal outcome. J Reprod Med 1980;24:191.
57. Cruikshank D (ed): Antepartum fetal surveillance. *Clin Obstet Gynecol* 1982;25:773–785.
58. Barrett J, Salyer SL, Boehm FH: The nonstress test: An evaluation of 1000 patients. *Am J Obstet Gynecol* 1981;141:153.
59. Schifrin BS, Foye G, Amato J, et al: Routine fetal heart rate monitoring in the antepartum period. *Obstet Gynecol* 1979;54:21.
60. Balfour HH, Block SH, Bowe ET, et al: Complications of fetal blood sampling. *Am J Obstet Gynecol* 1970;107:288.
61. Thadepalli H, Rambhatla K, Maidman JE, et al: Gonococcal sepsis secondary to fetal monitoring. *Am J Obstet Gynecol* 1976;126:510.
62. Overturf GD, Balfour G: Osteomyelitis and sepsis, severe complications of fetal monitoring. *Pediatrics* 1975;55:244.

63. Hall ML, Alexander CH: Fetal monitoring in a community hospital: Analysis of health maintenance organization, fee-for-service, and clinic populations. *Am J Obstet Gynecol* 1982;143:496.
64. Farb JF: Changing primary cesarean section patterns at a private hospital. *J Reprod Med* 1980;25:298.

CHAPTER 5

CESAREAN SECTION

Letitia K. Davis, ScD, EdM
Sharon L. Rosen, PhD

INTRODUCTION

Cesarean childbirth is widely accepted as an essential alternative to vaginal delivery which can, in many circumstances, reduce the risk of preventable handicap. The dramatic increase in the cesarean birth rate over the last 15 years, however, has prompted the concern of health care consumers and those responsible for burgeoning hospital costs, as well as the medical community. The increased use of cesarean surgery is highly controversial and a wide variety of opinions and strongly held beliefs about cesarean childbirth have been expressed. Proponents have stressed improvements in perinatal outcomes and the need to deliver infants with the least trauma possible.[1] Critics question whether it is the increased use of cesarean surgery that should be credited with the recent improvements in perinatal outcome and some have claimed that far too many cesareans are done unnecessarily or when they have become necessary because of medical interventions.[2] Research regarding the benefits and costs of increased reliance on cesarean surgery is inconclusive, and what constitutes an optimal cesarean birth rate, one which is neither too low nor too high, remains a subject of debate.[3,4]

Although the increased incidence of cesarean surgery has been widely accepted as one of several factors which have resulted in improved perinatal outcome, the benefits of cesarean childbirth, particularly those relating to infant morbidity and development, have not been well documented. Declining perinatal mortality rates over the last two decades are frequently interpreted as an indication that the increase in cesarean childbirth has improved perinatal health; however, this evidence is largely circumstantial. In fact, it is impossible to isolate the impact of the increased cesarean birth rate on perinatal mortality from concurrent changes such as the regionalization of perinatal care, dramatic advances in the care of neonates, the development of noninvasive techniques for evaluating fetal condition, dietary improvement, and the widespread availability of abortion and contraception. The most extensive research has been conducted on the use of cesarean delivery for breech presentation. Findings, however, are not consistent and the routine use of cesarean surgery in the case of breech presentation remains open to question.[5–7] In general, adequate epidemiologic and clinical investigations to systematically assess the extent to which cesarean birth results in improved perinatal health have not yet been undertaken.

On the other hand, the costs of cesarean childbirth are comparatively certain. While today a cesarean section is a basically safe operation, it remains a major surgical procedure, and women who give birth by cesarean are at much greater risk of childbirth-related illness or death than women who deliver vaginally. In addition to increased mortality and morbidity risks, there are added financial costs. The average cesarean birth has a length of stay double that of a normal vaginal delivery and may cost up to three times as much. Finally, the emotional costs of surgical childbirth to the mother, infant, and family, although not well studied, cannot be overlooked.[3,4]

While cesarean surgery is well recognized as an extremely valuable and essential obstetric procedure, the very rapid rise in cesarean birth rates without careful, scientific documentation of the benefits necessarily raises serious questions about its appropriate use. Concerns of the medical community about the escalating rates are widely cited in the literature. In 1976, when heads of teaching hospitals were asked to predict future cesarean birth rates, the majority estimated between 10 and 15% in 1981.[1] The national average for that year was 17.9%.[8] Those responsible for containing rapidly growing health care costs are scrutinizing cesarean birth rates on several counts. Not only is cesarean childbirth one of the ten most common surgical procedures, but investigators have consistently reported large differences in the cesarean birth rates among different hospitals.[3,4]

In 1979, the National Institutes of Health initiated a consensus development process which brought together representatives from different disciplines, including biomedical research scientists, practicing physicians, and consumers, to assess the efficacy and appropriateness of the trend toward increased reliance on cesarean childbirth. While information sufficient to determine an optimal cesarean birth rate was not found to exist, the consensus task force concluded that the spiraling cesarean birth rate could be "stopped and perhaps reversed while continuing to make improvements in maternal and fetal outcomes."[3]

We shall review in the first part of this chapter the epidemiologic literature on cesarean birth in the United States and, in the second part, present the results of a detailed analysis of delivery methods in Massachusetts during 1981.

NATIONAL EXPERIENCE AND TRENDS IN CESAREAN DELIVERY

Prior to 1965, a cesarean delivery was a relatively infrequent event, with only 2–5% of births being delivered by cesarean. Between 1965 and 1975, the United States cesarean

Table 5-1
Cesarean Section Rates for Nonfederal Short-stay Hospitals in the United States and the Northeast, 1970–1981*

Year	United States	Northeast
1970	5.5	6.2
1971	5.8	7.4
1972	7.0	7.3
1973	8.0	9.0
1974	9.2	10.8
1975	10.4	11.9
1976	12.1	14.6
1977	13.7	15.9
1978	15.2	17.6
1979	16.4	18.1
1980	16.5	19.2
1981	17.9	20.0
1982	18.5	19.1
1983	20.3	21.5

*From Placek PJ, Taffel SM: Trends in cesarean section rates for the United States, 1970–1978. *Public Health Rep* 1980;95:540–548,[10] and additional National Hospital Discharge Survey data, National Center for Health Statistics.

section rate (defined as the number of cesarean deliveries per 100 deliveries) rose from 4.5 to 10.4, and recently published data indicate that the United States cesarean section rate for 1983 was 20.3 (Table 5-1).[8,9] This represents more than a quadrupling of the rate in an 18-year period. The rapid increase in cesarean section rates has been observed in all areas of the country and in various subgroupings of the population, reflecting a broad-based change in obstetric practice. During the same period, cesarean delivery rates have also increased in other countries with comparable medical resources and health needs, notably Canada, France, Great Britain, Norway, and the Netherlands. The rate of change, however, has varied in different countries, with the United States experiencing the sharpest increase.[3] On a regional basis within the United

States, the rates since 1970 have consistently been highest in the New England states.[9,10]

A variety of factors have been suggested as contributors to the steadily rising trend. Changing expectations about pregnancy outcomes and an increasing emphasis on delivering infants free of preventable handicaps have been widely cited as contributing factors. Some have described this as an increased emphasis on delivering the "perfect baby," in a society where there is greater choice about childbearing and fewer children per family. Reluctance to accept the risks to both infant and mother which are associated with midforceps deliveries is also a factor, and cesareans, to a large extent, have replaced vaginal deliveries previously accomplished by midforceps. The introduction of new medical technologies, in particular the fetal heart monitor, which electronically measures the fetal heart rate, has also been cited as a cause for the rising cesarean birth rate, as have changes in maternal age and parity. Increases in obstetric specialization and training programs which emphasize intervention-oriented obstetrics have been suggested as contributors as well. Changing expectations about pregnancy outcome and the availability of new technologies both reflect and contribute to the current medicolegal climate, and the increased reliance on cesarean surgery has also been attributed to the growing tendency to practice "defensive medicine." In a 1979 survey, Marieskind found fear of malpractice suits the most frequent reason given by physicians for the increase in cesarean births.[4] Economic incentives have also been suggested as determinants. Many health insurance plans have offered more extensive coverage for cesarean births, and the added length of stay for cesareans may be financially attractive to hospitals, particularly in light of the declining birth rate and resultant empty obstetrical beds.[3,4]

The standard practice to surgically deliver all pregnant women who have had previous cesareans is also a large factor in the rising rates. The policy of routine "repeats" has inevitably led to a rise in the overall rate as women who have had primary cesareans became pregnant again. "Once a cesarean, always a cesarean" has been the obstetrical norm in the United States since the early 1900s. However, a number of recent investigations have demonstrated that large proportions of women with previous cesareans have had subsequent successful vaginal deliveries, and in Western Europe, many obstetrical practices plan a trial of labor for the majority of patients with previous cesareans.[3] The necessity of routine repeat cesareans is currently being questioned in this country as well. While a reversal of the repeat cesarean policy may be predicted for the future, routine repeat cesareans have unquestionably contributed to the rising cesarean birth rates observed in the United States over the last several decades.[3,10,11]

No single factor can be identified as causing the increase in cesarean births. For example, changing expectations about pregnancy outcomes cannot be understood in isolation from changing technologies, while in turn, changing expectations may be an impetus for technologic advance. Rather, a number of complex, interacting factors have combined to shape modern obstetric practice, and it is difficult to evaluate empirically the impact of these many factors on the cesarean delivery rate. A number of studies, however, have been undertaken relating cesarean delivery to maternal and health care characteristics. Major findings reported in the literature are discussed below.

CESAREAN POPULATION

Investigators have examined birth rates in relation to a variety of maternal characteristics in order to identify the populations at greatest risk of cesarean delivery. Maternal age and infant birth weight have been found to be the strongest predictors of cesarean birth.

Maternal Age

Studies have consistently shown that the risk of cesarean delivery is higher among older women, with women 30 years or older frequently found to be two to three times as likely to have cesareans as women less than 20 years old.[3,4,10,19] Dysfunctional labor and malpresentation, both indications for cesarean surgery, have been reported to be twice as common in older women.[4] Marieskind also suggested that the management of labor may be different in older women, referring to one study which found a higher incidence of sedation in the older maternal population.[4]

An increasing proportion of women in the United States are having their first child when they are older. This demographic shift has been suggested as a factor in the rising cesarean birth rate. Several studies of cesarean trends by age, however, have shown that the cesarean delivery rate has increased much more rapidly for younger women than for older women over the last several decades. Placek et al reported that the increase in the national rate from 1965 to 1981 has been threefold for women over 30 years old whereas it has been greater than fourfold for women under 30.[9] The increase in average maternal age, therefore, cannot alone account for the rising trend. The sharp rise in rates for younger women may lead to still higher overall rates in the future if the current norm of "once a cesarean, always a cesarean" generally prevails and these women have additional deliveries.

Infant Birth Weight

Infant birth weight is also a strong predictor of cesarean birth. Mothers giving birth to infants in the favorable weight range of 2500–4000 g have consistently been found to be less likely to deliver by cesarean than women delivering lighter or heavier weight infants. Women delivering very small infants (less than 1000 g) may be an exception, as several investigators have shown infants in this category more likely to be delivered vaginally.[3] Data from New York City and California indicate that rates have risen most sharply for infants weighing less than 1500 g, possibly reflecting the increased use of cesarean surgery to deliver compromised infants as atraumatically as possible. Since less than 1% of all babies are in this weight category, however, the contribution of any sharp rise in this group to the overall rate is extremely small.[3] Other investigators have shown similar rates of increase for all birth weights.[3,13]

An increase in the average birth weight over the last 20 years has been offered as one explanation for the overall rise in cesarean births in that mothers of heavier infants are more likely to be diagnosed with cephalopelvic disproportion, an indication for cesarean surgery. This suggestion has not been borne out by the data, however, which indicate that the average infant birth weight increased less than two ounces between 1966 and 1976, a period when the cesarean delivery rate doubled.[4]

Prenatal Care

Studies of the adequacy of prenatal care obtained by mothers and the relation of this factor to cesarean birth have differed in their findings. Studies of births in California and New York City revealed that women who received less prenatal care had lower cesarean section rates; however, other differences between the prenatal care groups, such as age and parity, were not taken into account in these investigations.[3,14] Williams and Hawes[15] reported lower cesarean section rates in hospitals serving greater proportions of women with no prenatal care, yet Placek,[16] in an analysis of National Natality Survey data for 1972, found no association between prenatal care and cesarean birth.[15,16] Zdeb et al found lower cesarean section rates in women beginning prenatal care later, but this association disappeared when other differences beween prenatal care groups were accounted for in the analysis.[17] While these findings are inconsistent, they do suggest that what has, in some cases, appeared as a positive relationship between cesarean birth and less prenatal care in simple analyses did not persist when potential confounding factors were taken into account.

Marital Status

Several studies have noted differences in cesarean birth rates based on marital status. Placek et al reported slightly higher rates for married women in both 1970 and 1978 in their analysis of data from the National Hospital Discharge Survey.[9] These same authors found no significant difference in the cesarean section rates for married and unmarried women based on data from the 1980 National Natality Survey.[12] Williams and Hawes found higher rates in hospitals serving greater proportions of married women.[15] Zdeb et al found slightly higher rates for married women, even after taking maternal age and parity into account.[17]

Maternal Residence

Differences in cesarean birth rates based on maternal residence have also been reported. In the 1972 National Natality Study, 8.3% of metropolitan women were delivered by cesarean in contrast to 5.2% of nonmetropolitan women.[16] Williams and Chen[13] reported that rural hospitals in California had lower rates than urban hospitals. This finding could, however, be attributed to referrals of high-risk pregnancies to urban hospitals. Higher cesarean birth rates for metropolitan women may reflect the fact that there are more diverse, higher-risk populations residing in urban areas. They may also be explained by the greater availability of obstetric technologies in the larger hospitals and teaching institutions more prevalent in urban areas.

Maternal Education and Ethnicity

It has been suggested, both implicitly and explicitly, that a mother's socioeconomic status may affect her likelihood of having a cesarean birth. As cesarean surgery is a comparatively expensive procedure requiring a more sophisticated level of obstetric care, and because the quest for the "perfect baby" is generally attributed to more affluent sectors of the population, one might predict that women of higher socioeconomic status are more likely to deliver by cesarean. Alternatively, women of lower socioeconomic status tend to have more medical risk factors and, therefore, may be more likely to have cesarean births. Available findings on the association between economic status and cesarean birth are inconclusive.

Information on cesarean birth and annual family income was collected in the National Natality Survey conducted in 1972 and again in 1980 by the National Center for Health Statistics. In the analysis of 1972 data, cesarean sections were found to be performed more often on women with high incomes.[16] Recently published findings based on the 1980 data revealed no significant association between income and the cesarean section rate after adjusting for maternal age and parity.[12]

Education is a widely accepted indicator of socioeconomic status. Several studies have revealed increasing cesarean birth rates with increasing level of maternal education, implying a greater likelihood of cesarean birth in women of higher socioeconomic status. In these studies, however, maternal age, which is strongly correlated with both education and cesarean birth, was not taken into account.[3,16] When age and other confounding factors were controlled for in the study by Zdeb et al, women with less education were actually found to have higher cesarean section rates.[17] Data from the 1980 National Natality Study reveal no significant association between education and the cesarean section rate after adjustments are made for maternal age.[12]

Race or ethnicity is frequently considered another indicator of socioeconomic status to the extent that it is correlated with socioeconomic level. Several investigators have reported differences by race, but these findings are not consistent. In the 1972 National Natality Survey, cesarean rates were found to be higher for nonwhites (9.4) than for whites (7.0).[16] Placek and Taffel found that the relationship between cesarean birth and race varied by region of the country. Rates were higher for whites in the South but slightly higher for nonwhites in the West and Northeast.[10] Data from Baltimore hospitals revealed higher cesarean birth rates for blacks.[18] In a study of births in New York City, only minor differences were found by race and ethnic group. However, within the very-low-birth-weight class (less than 1500 g), blacks had lower cesarean birth rates than whites.[3] Williams and Hawes found lower cesarean section rates in California hospitals serving greater proportions of Spanish-surname mothers.[15] In a more recent California study, rates were higher for blacks than for whites independent of maternal age, infant birth weight, and parity.[13] Alternatively, Placek and Taffel, in their analysis of the 1980 National Natality Survey data, found higher cesarean section rates for whites after taking age and parity into account.[12] These varied findings on race may reflect differences in methods of data collection and analysis. They may also indicate that the relationship between cesarean birth and race may differ with location and may vary over time.

HEALTH SYSTEM FACTORS

In addition to the characteristics of the maternal population, incentives operating within the health care system have been suggested as factors contributing to the rise in cesarean birth rates. Investigators have examined cesarean births in relation to a variety of hospital characteristics in order to assess the potential associations between health system factors and delivery methods. The findings are generally inconsistent, and firm conclusions regarding the impact of health systems factors on cesarean birth rates cannot be drawn.

Hospital Teaching Status

It has been suggested that the teaching status of hospitals might be related to cesarean birth rates, where teaching programs emphasize both intervention-oriented obstetrics and the need to provide physicians-in-training clinical experience in performing cesareans.[3] Several studies have shown that cesarean delivery rates are higher in teaching hospitals than in nonteaching hospitals. However, factors such as potential differences in populations served by these hospitals were not controlled for in deriving these results.[17,19] It is difficult to assess the relationship between teaching status and delivery methods because teaching hospitals frequently differ from nonteaching hospitals in other ways which may also account for differences in cesarean birth rates. Teaching hospitals, for example, are generally larger and located in urban settings, serving higher-risk populations. Williams and Hawes found no independent association between cesarean birth rates and teaching hospitals when other factors were controlled for in the analysis.[15] In a recent study, Williams and Chen found that teaching hospitals in California had lower cesarean section rates than expected based on the statewide experience over a three-year period.[13]

Hospital Size

Findings on the association between cesarean birth and hospital size also vary. A number of studies have revealed that cesarean birth rates are higher in larger hospitals.[4] Taffel and coworkers observed increasing rates with increasing hospital size in the nation as a whole, but they did not observe this trend in the Northeast.[8,9] Williams and Chen recently reported that rates in very large and very small hospitals were less than expected.[13] In 1978, Baskett predicted a rise in the cesarean birth rates for large hospitals and static or falling rates in smaller hospitals as "it becomes unacceptable to perform cesareans without adequate personnel," but this prediction has not been borne out in the literature.[20]

Availability of Neonatal Intensive Care

Hospitals with neonatal intensive care units, which are frequently the larger teaching hospitals, would be predicted to have higher ccsarean delivery rates as they serve as tertiary referral centers for high-risk pregnancies. However, little information is available on the relationship between a hospital's level of obstetric care and cesarean birth. Surprisingly, in a recent California study, tertiary-care hospitals were found to have lower cesarean section rates than hospitals providing only primary and secondary level care.[13]

Obstetric Specialization

Increases in obstetric specialization have been cited as another cause of rising cesarean birth rates on the grounds that specialized training promotes a wider range of choices of procedures. In the United States, the percentage of births delivered by specialists rose from 68% in 1968 to 81% in 1977.[3] During this time period, the cesarean section rate rose from 5.0 to 13.7. Similar positive correlations between cesarean section rates and obstetric specialization have been observed in a number of Western European countries, but this evidence must be viewed as circumstantial and does not establish a causal link between cesarean birth and obstetric specialization.[3] A more direct finding is the documented positive association between hospital-specific cesarean section rates and percent of deliveries by specialists in the Williams and Hawes study of California births.[15] This association was observed even after controlling for other factors such as maternal age and parity.[15]

Hospital Ownership

Economic incentives have also been cited as an explanation for the increase in cesarean births.[3,4] If monetary factors are important determinants, cesarean section rates might be expected to vary by hospital ownership, as proprietary hospitals have incentives to perform procedures that lengthen stay and increase the utilization of resources which represent high capital investments. Placek et al, in their analysis of data from nonfederal, short-stay hospitals for 1981, observed the highest cesarean birth rates in proprietary hospitals, followed by nonprofit hospitals and government hospitals.[9] They observed a similar rank for short-stay hospitals in the nation as a whole and in the Northeast over the past decade.[10] These findings, however, have not been supported in other investigations. In New York City, nonprofit and proprietary hospitals were found to have similar rates, and Williams and Hawes found a significant positive association between cesarean section rates and nonprofit but not proprietary ownership.[3,15] On the basis of these inconsistent findings, it is doubtful that the type of hospital ownership is an important determinant of cesarean delivery rates.

Insurance Coverage

The possibility that economic considerations influence cesarean birth rates raises questions about the influence of insurance coverage and various methods of health care cost reimbursement on cesarean section rates. Women without health insurance coverage might be expected to experience lower cesarean delivery rates than women with health insurance, given that surgical delivery generally involves higher total medical charges. The issue of insurance coverage has been complicated by the fact that, in the past, many individual and group insurance plans discriminated between vaginal and cesarean deliveries. These plans frequently offer extensive coverage for cesarean births while limiting coverage following vaginal delivery.[3] Under the 1978 amendments to the civil rights law, however, employers have been required to provide similar health insurance benefits for vaginal and cesarean deliveries.[21] Cesarean delivery rates might also be expected to be lower among women covered by prepaid health plans, particularly in the case of hospitals owned by health maintenance organizations (HMOs).

Findings on insurance coverage and cesarean delivery rates must be interpreted with caution, as there are differences other than type of insurance between women with different insurance plans. Placek et al[9] found higher cesarean section rates in 1980 and 1981 for women with Blue Cross or other private insurance, based on nationwide data. However, other differences between women with and without private insurance which might also account for the findings were not taken into account in computing these rates. In the 1980 data, for example, older married and white women were found to be more likely to have Blue Cross or other private insurance than young, single, and nonwhite women.[22] In an analysis of births in New York City, women with private insurance were found to have the highest cesarean section rates, whereas Medicaid patients had the lowest rates.[3] Rates were also lower for Medicaid recipients in California in 1977 than for the state as a whole. Again, other differences between insurance groups were not taken into account in deriving these results.[3] In a Boston study, the primary cesarean section rate was lower for members of an HMO than for fee-for-service patients delivered at the same hospital.[23] Williams and Hawes found that cesarean section rates were lower for women covered by the Kaiser prepaid health plan even after controlling for other differences; they suggested that "prepayment has an independent, attenuating impact on the rate of surgical intervention."[15]

COMPLICATIONS IN CESAREAN DELIVERIES

The steady rise in cesarean birth rates has prompted a number of investigators to examine the various maternal and fetal complications associated with cesarean deliveries. One of the most striking findings is the increase in the proportion of all deliveries with reported complications. Based on a national sample of hospital discharge data collected by the Commission on Professional and Hospital Activities (CPHA), the proportion of all deliveries with complications increased from 30.1% in 1970 to 45.6% in 1978.[3] In a study of births in New York City, 88.1% of all births had no reported complications in 1968–1969 whereas only 74.0% of all births were free of complications in 1976–1977.[3] Taffel and Placek recently reported an increase in deliveries with one or more stated complication from 17.6% in 1970 to approximately half (49.9%) of all deliveries in 1980.[24] Different schemes have been used for classifying complications in the abovementioned studies, and quantitative comparisons of the various study results are not appropriate. The data, however, strongly indicate that an increasing proportion of women are being reported to have complications of labor and delivery. It has been suggested that this increase is due mainly to diagnostic changes and changes in reporting, which reflect, in large part, earlier recognition of pathology, rather than alterations in the prevalence of complications.

According to the data provided by CPHA, four complications accounted for approximately 80% of all cesareans in 1978: dystocia (31% of all cesarean deliveries); previous cesarean (31%); breech presentation (12%); and fetal distress

(5%).[3] Other investigators have also identified these same four complications as the most frequently reported indications for cesarean birth in recent years.[3,24]

Changes in both the complication-specific cesarean birth rates and in the percentage of births diagnosed with complications will contribute to changes in the overall cesarean birth rate. Consider the findings for CPHA hospitals reported in Table 5-2. While the proportion of all deliveries that were breech presentation remained relatively constant (approximately 3%) between 1970 and 1978, the cesarean delivery rate for breech presentation rose from 11.6 to 60.1 during this same time period. National data reviewed by Taffel and Placek reveal a similar increase in the complication-specific rate, indicating a dramatic shift in the management of breech presentations.[24] In contrast, the management of previous cesareans has remained constant, with over 98% of all women with previous cesareans delivering by repeat cesarean throughout the decade. The percentage of deliveries by women with previous cesareans in the nation as a whole, however, increased from 2.1 in 1970 to 4.6 in 1978, reflecting the increase in the primary cesarean rate.[3]

The data provided by CPHA were also analyzed to identify which complications contributed most heavily to the overall rise in the cesarean delivery rate from 1970 to 1978. As shown in Table 5-3, dystocia was identified as the largest contributor, followed by previous cesarean, other fetal complications (which included fetal distress), and breech presentation. For dystocia and other fetal complications, the major contribution was attributable to substantial increases in making these diagnoses, although the cesarean delivery rates for these complications also increased. For women with previous cesareans, virtually all the contribution was due to the increase in the percentage of women with this diagnosis. Conversely, for breech presentations, virtually all its contribution was due to an increase in the use of cesarean delivery for this complication. An analysis of New York City births

Table 5-2
Cesarean Delivery Rate (CDR) by Complication and Percent of All Deliveries Having Each Complication, 1970 and 1978*

	CDR†		Percent with complication	
Complication	*1970*	*1978*	*1970*	*1978*
No mention	0.2	0.2	69.9	54.4
Lacerations	0.0	0.1	9.8	11.8
Previous cesarean	98.3	98.9	2.1	4.6
Dystocia‡	50.6	67.0	3.8	6.7
Breech	11.6	60.1	2.9	2.8
Persistent occiput posterior	3.5	10.3	1.4	1.2
Other malpresentations	30.5	37.2	0.8	1.0
Other "maternal"§	38.2	50.5	1.4	1.2
Other "fetal"‖	6.3	25.5	2.8	8.0
Other, unspecified	6.1	7.0	5.2	8.3
All	5.7	14.7	100.0	100.0

*Based on a national sample of hospital discharge data collected by the Commission on Professional Activities, reported in *Cesarean Childbirth*, US Department of Health and Human Services, NIH Publication No. 82-2067, October 1981.[3]
†Cesarean deliveries per 100 total deliveries.
‡Fetopelvic disproportion, abnormal pelvis, prolonged labor.
§Antepartum hemorrhage, prior gynecologic surgery.
‖Premature rupture of membrane, premature labor, multiple pregnancy, prolonged ROM, prolonged pregnancy, fetal distress.

Table 5-3
Complication-specific Contribution to Rise in Cesarean Delivery Rate (CDR) from 1970 to 1978*

	Percent contribution to rise		
Complication	*From CDR change*	*From % change in diagnosis*	*Total*
No mention	0.0	0.0	0.0
Lacerations	0.0	1.1	1.1
Previous cesarean section	0.0	27.0	27.0
Dystocia†	6.7	22.5	29.2
Breech	15.7	0.0	15.7
Persistent occiput posterior	1.1	0.0	1.1
Other malpresentations	1.1	1.1	2.2
Other "maternal"‡	2.3	−1.1	1.2
Other "fetal"§	5.6	14.6	20.2
Other, unspecified	0.0	2.3	2.3
All	32.5	67.5	100.0‖

*Based on a national sample of hospital discharge data collected by the Commission on Professional and Hospital Activities reported in *Cesarean Childbirth*, US Department of Health and Human Services, NIH Publication No. 82-2067, October 1981.[3]
†Fetopelvic disproportion, abnormal pelvis, prolonged labor.
‡Antepartum hemorrhage, prior gynecologic surgery.
§PROM, premature labor, multiple pregnancy, prolonged rupture of membranes, prolonged pregnancy, fetal distress.
‖Percents not equal 100.0 due to rounding.

during 1968–1969 and 1976–1977 also revealed dystocia, previous cesareans, breech, and fetal distress as the largest contributors to the rising cesarean birth rate.[3]

The lack of uniformity in classifying complications of labor and delivery has made it difficult to identify trends in complications over time and to compare the results of various studies. There are consistencies in the available data, however, which enable some conclusions to be drawn. The cesarean birth rate has increased dramatically for breech presentations, reflecting a change in obstetrical management of this complication. More women are presenting with previous cesareans which may be attributed to the rise in the primary cesarean birth rate. More women are also being diagnosed with fetal distress and dystocia. In several studies, increases in the frequency of diagnoses of fetal distress have been correlated with the increasing use of electronic fetal heart monitors, and it is suggested that the use of fetal heart monitors has resulted in increased numbers of cesareans performed for fetal distress.[3,25,26] Alternatively, Neutra et al have documented a reduction in cesareans for fetal distress with the introduction of fetal heart monitoring and better information about the infant.[27] The use of fetal heart monitors, which may restrict a woman's movement during labor, may also play a role in other complications associated with cesarean delivery such as failure to progress in labor. The impact of electronic fetal heart monitoring on the cesarean delivery rate and on fetal outcome remains controversial.

The reasons for the large increase in the frequency of the diagnosis of dystocia are less well understood. Dystocia is a broad term encompassing a heterogeneous group of patients whose progress in labor is unsatisfactory due to a variety of factors including a poorly shaped pelvis, a large infant, and inadequate uterine contractions. The diagnosis of dystocia involves subjective judgement, however, and it has been suggested that the increased use of this diagnosis reflects a change in the attitude of obstetricians toward what constitutes a reasonable duration of labor.

SUMMARY

In summary, the steady increase in cesarean births in this country has been consistently observed across various subgroups of the population in numerous investigations. The data on complications of labor and delivery and cesarean births reveal major shifts in obstetric practice and suggest that the increased cesarean birth rate has been more heavily affected by changes in the diagnosis and management of medical complications than by any changes in the physiological characteristics of the pregnant population.

Numerous investigators have examined cesarean birth rates in relation to a variety of maternal and health care characteristics in an effort to identify predictors of cesarean delivery. Maternal age and infant birth weight have consistently been identified as the strongest risk factors for cesarean birth, with older women and women delivering infants outside of the favorable weight range being more likely to give birth by cesarean. Women residing in metropolitan areas have also generally been found at greater risk of cesarean delivery. Findings regarding the relationship between cesarean birth and maternal race and ethnicity, education, marital status, and adequacy of care are inconsistent, as are findings regarding the relationship between cesarean delivery and various health system characteristics.

The interpretation of the findings regarding predictors of cesarean birth is made difficult by the many complex, interacting factors. Some of the inconsistencies between studies may be accounted for by different methods of data analysis, in particular differences between simple and multivariate techniques. Others likely reflect changes in predictors of cesarean birth over time, as a once comparatively uncommon surgical procedure has become a routine obstetrical practice. Given the physical, emotional, and financial costs of cesarean delivery and its still largely uncertain benefits, further research is needed to clarify the determinants of cesarean delivery and the impact of cesarean birth on maternal and infant health.

CESAREAN BIRTHS IN MASSACHUSETTS

In July 1980, an item was added to the Massachusetts birth certificate distinguishing vaginal from cesarean deliveries. This change in data collection enabled the Department of Public Health to utilize, for the first time, vital records for the study of cesarean births in Massachusetts. The department conducted a detailed analysis of delivery methods in Massachusetts during fiscal year 1981 (July 1, 1980–June 30, 1981).[28] The study population was limited to 31,876 first, live resident births. Cesarean birth rates were examined in relation to a variety of maternal and hospital characteristics using descriptive and multivariate methods. Hospital-specific rates were also examined and the variability in hospital-specific rates explored using multiple regression techniques. The major findings of the study are summarized below.

1. Older women and women delivering low- or heavy-birth-weight infants in Massachusetts were more likely to give birth by cesarean. Cesarean birth rates were highest for women delivering infants between 1001 and 1500 g.

2. Maternal age was strongly correlated with a number of other previously reported predictors of cesarean birth such as maternal race and education and adequacy of prenatal care. Differences between crude and age-adjusted rates revealed the importance of taking patient risk factors such as maternal age into account in studying delivery methods.

3. Women with less education were found to be more likely to give birth by cesarean when maternal age was taken into account. This result contradicts prevailing findings that cesarean birth rates increase with maternal education but is consistent with results reported by Zdeb et al, who also accounted for maternal age in their analysis of delivery methods in New York State.[17]

4. There was a suggestion in the data that Hispanics were more likely to give birth by cesarean than either black or non-Hispanic white women. These findings were based on small numbers, however, and were therefore difficult to interpret. Older black women were found to have very high cesarean birth rates.

5. The findings regarding maternal education and race raise the possibility that women of lower socioeconomic status are more likely to deliver by cesarean than women of higher socioeconomic levels in Massachusetts. Possible explanations for such an association include differences in social risk factors, such as nutritional status, and equity of care considerations which could not be addressed in this study.

6. Both women who lived in the greater Boston area (Health Service Area IV) and women who gave birth in the greater Boston area were more likely to deliver by cesarean than women who lived and women who gave birth in other parts of Massachusetts. These associations were revealed consistently throughout the report and appeared to be independent of regional differences in maternal age, race, infant birth weight, hospital teaching status, or the availability of neonatal intensive care.

7. Findings regarding the relationship between cesarean birth and hospital characteristics are difficult to interpret due to multiple correlations between hospital characteristics such as size, teaching status, and availability of neonatal intensive care. In general, the study revealed strikingly few associations between cesarean birth and hospital characteristics. Most notably, neither teaching status nor the presence of a neonatal intensive care unit had independent associations with cesarean birth when other factors were controlled for in the analysis. These findings suggested that cesarean surgery is performed routinely across the variety of hospital settings in Massachusetts.

8. Hospital-specific rates were highly variable, ranging from 0 to 31.4, with a weighted average of 18.5. With a single exception, the 10 hospitals with the highest rates did not have neonatal intensive care units to which high-risk pregnancies are likely referred. Less than 30% of the variability in hospital-specific rates could be explained by the leading factors known to be associated with cesarean delivery, including differences in the maternal age and infant birth weight distributions of

the hospital's patient populations or in the availability of neonatal intensive care. Additional factors not accounted for in the analysis, such as other patient risk factors, physician-specific practices, and hospital policies regarding cesarean birth, must therefore contribute to the variation in hospital-specific cesarean birth rates.

REFERENCES

1. Jones OH: Cesarean section in present-day obstetrics. Presidential address. *Am J Obstet Gynecol* 1976;126:521–530.
2. Cohen NW, Esther LD: *Silent Knife, Cesarean Prevention and Vaginal Birth After Cesarean.* South Hadley, Massachusetts, Bergun and Garvey, 1983.
3. *Cesarean Childbirth.* US Department of Health and Human Services, Public Health Service, National Institutes of Health, NIH Publication No 82-2067, October 1981.
4. Marieskind HI: *An Evaluation of Cesarean Section in the United States.* Office of the Assistant Secretary for Planning and Evaluation/Health, Department of Health, Education and Welfare, June 1979.
5. Russell JK: Breech: Vaginal delivery or cesarean section? *Br Med J* 1982;285:830–831.
6. Main DM, Main EK, Maurer MM: Cesarean section versus vaginal delivery for the breech fetus weighing less than 1,500 grams. *Am J Obstet Gynecol* 1983;146:580–584.
7. Effer SB, Saigal S, Rand C, et al: Effect of delivery method on outcomes in the very low birth weight breech infant: Is the improved survival related to cesarean section or other perinatal care maneuvers? *Am J Obstet Gynecol* 1983;145:123–128.
8. Taffel SM, Placek PJ: One fifth of 1983 US births by cesarean section. *Am J Public Health* 1985;75:190.
9. Placek PJ, Taffel S, Moien M: Cesarean section delivery rates: United States, 1981. *Am J Public Health* 1983;73:861–862.
10. Placek PJ, Taffel SM: Trends in cesarean section rates for the United States, 1970–1978. *Public Health Rep* 1980;95:540–548.
11. Minkoff HL, Schwarz RH: The rising cesarean section rate: Can it safely be reversed? *Obstet Gynecol* 1980;56:135–143.
12. Placek PJ, Taffel SM, Keppel KG: Maternal and infant characteristics associated with cesarean section delivery, in *Health,*

United States, US Dept of Health and Human Services publication No. (PHS)84-1232. Government Printing Office, 1983.

13. Williams RL, Chen PM: Controlling the rise in cesarean section rates by the dissemination of information from vital records. *Am J Public Health* 1983;73:863–867.
14. Petitti D, Olson RO, Williams RL: Cesarean section in California— 1960 through 1975. *Am J Obstet Gynecol* 1979;133:391–397.
15. Williams RL, Hawes WE: Cesarean section, fetal monitoring and perinatal mortality in California. *Am J Public Health* 1979;69: 864–870.
16. Placek PJ: *Type of Delivery Associated With Social, Demographic, Maternal Health, Infant Health and Health Insurance Factors.* Findings from the 1972 US National Natality Survey, Proceedings of the Social Statistics Section, 1977, Part II. Washington, DC, American Statistical Association, 1978.
17. Zdeb MS, Therriault GD, Logrillo VM: Cesarean sections in upstate New York, 1968–1978. *Am J Epidemiol* 1980;112:395–403.
18. Gibbons LK: *Analysis of The Rise in C-Section in Baltimore.* Doctoral dissertation, School of Hygiene and Public Health, The Johns Hopkins University, 1976.
19. Lowe JA, Klassen DF, Loup RJ: Cesarean sections in United States PAS hospitals. *PAS Reporter* 1976;14:1–55.
20. Baskett TF: Cesarean section: What is an acceptable rate? *Can Med Assoc J* 1978;118:1019–1020.
21. Amendments to Title VII of the Civil Rights Act of 1964, PL 95-555, 1978.
22. Keppel KG, Taffel SH, Placek PJ: *Source of Hospital Payment of Deliveries in the United States,* 1980. Paper presented at the Annual Meeting of the American Public Health Association, Montreal, Canada, November, 1982.
23. Wilner SI, Monson RR, Schoenbaum SC, et al: A comparison of the quality of maternity care between a health maintenance organization and fee for services practices. *N Engl J Med* 1981;304(13): 784–787.
24. Taffel SM, Placek PJ: Complications in cesarean and non-cesarean deliveries, United States, 1980. *Am J Public Health* 1983;73:856–860.
25. Banta HD, Thacker SB: *Costs and Benefits of Electronic Fetal Monitoring: A Review of the Literature.* NCHSR Research Report Series, US Department of Public Health, Education and

Welfare, Public Health Service, DHEW Publication No (PHS) 79-3245, April, 1979.

26. Placek PJ, Keppel KG, Taffel SM, et al: Electronic fetal monitoring in relation to cesarean section delivery, for live births and stillbirths in the US, 1980. *Public Health Rep* 1984;99:173–183.
27. Neutra RR, Greenland S, Friedman EA: The effect of fetal monitoring on C-section rates. *Obstet Gynecol* 1980;55:175.
28. Davis LK, Rosen SL, Hannan MT, et al: *Cesarean Birth in Massachusetts.* Boston, Department of Public Health, Commonwealth of Massachusetts, 1984.

CHAPTER 6

REPRODUCTIVE OUTCOME OF THE OLDER GRAVIDA

David Acker, MD
Benjamin P. Sachs, MB.BS, DPH(C)

INTRODUCTION

The Old Testament relates the birth of Isaac to Abraham and Sarah (Genesis 17:17). Sarah was reported to be 91 years old at the time of her pregnancy. In her conversations with God, Sarah was concerned about her husband's old age and his effect on her fertility and reproductive outcome. God, however, in the interest of marital harmony, reports to Abraham that Sarah is concerned with her own advancing years. In spite of advanced maternal and paternal age, the result was satisfactory. At age 91, there was no doubt that Sarah was an elderly gravida; however, confusion over the definition of the term elderly primigravida persisted until the Council of the International Federation of Obstetricians and Gynecologists (CIFOG) in 1958 determined that at age 35 a primigravida becomes elderly. There is no agreed upon, or arbitrarily assigned, age that designates a multigravida elderly.

In the current decade, due mainly to an expected increase in the number of women aged 35–44, more babies can be expected to be born to older women (although none would be expected to be as old as Sarah) than in the previous decade.[1]

Hypertension and diabetes mellitus play a crucial role in determining the maternal and fetal outcome in the pregnancies of older gravidas. This chapter will first review the relationship between pregnancy outcome and these two common serious medical complications and then review recent obstetrical literature relating to the maternal and fetal risks posed by pregnancy conceived later in reproductive life.

HYPERTENSION

A clear understanding of the relationship of hypertension, advanced maternal age, and pregnancy outcome necessitates a review of the management and the perinatal outcome of pregnancy complicated by both chronic and acute hypertension. The Collaborative Perinatal Project (CCP), under the auspices of the National Institute of Neurological and Communicative Disorders and Strokes prospectively collected data from 12 urban institutions on 38,636 gravidas who carried single fetuses, were seen prior to the 28th week of their pregnancy, and had at least four antenatal visits.[2] The data base included 269,668 blood pressure recordings in addition to a similar number of recordings related to the presence or absence of edema, weight gain, and degree of proteinuria. Although patients were originally grouped according to race, age, and parity, the results were comparable and the data were therefore pooled. The perinatal outcome was directly and additively related to both elevation in blood pressure and the presence of proteinuria. Even a slight elevation of diastolic blood pressure to 85 mm Hg (and slight proteinuria) was associated with a sevenfold increase in the perinatal mortality compared to the normotensive patient without proteinuria. The same slightly elevated diastolic blood pressure associated with 2+ or greater proteinuria increased the perinatal mortality by a factor of 10. An elevation in the diastolic pressure to >94 mm Hg increased perinatal mortality by a factor of

4. If even slight (trace to 1+) proteinuria was also present, perinatal mortality increased by a factor of 20. Although hypertensive gravidas represented slightly less than 1/7 of the total patient population, their pregnancies were associated with 1/3 of the stillborns.

The cause of death was ascertained by autopsy in 80% of the losses.[3] The excess mortality in the pregnancies complicated by hypertension was due to the following conditions: (1) Large placental infarcts (defined as infarcts greater than 3 cm noted in greater than 25% of the placentae) accounted for 42% of excess mortality. (2) Placental growth retardation (defined as placental weight less than the 40th percentile) accounted for 15% of excess mortality. (3) Abruptio placentae (defined by the usual clinical/laboratory criteria) accounted for 13% of excess mortality.

Unfortunately appreciation of the risk and an understanding of the pathological changes is not synonymous with successful or even noncontroversial methods of management. Even the utility of antihypertensive medication during pregnancy remains controversial. Sabii et al described 211 patients delivered at the E.H. Crump Women's Hospital in Memphis, Tennessee.[4] All patients had a documented history of chronic hypertension before pregnancy and at least two blood pressure readings of ≥140/90 mm Hg within the hospital. Only 36 of the 211 patients were considered ill enough to have had antihypertensive medication offered to them prior to their current pregnancy, and all had their medication discontinued upon enrollment in the antenatal clinic.

The patients were then followed closely during frequent antenatal visits. The 211 women experienced 215 births (four sets of twins), two stillborns and four neonatal deaths, yielding a perinatal mortality rate (PMR) of 27.9/1000 live births. All losses occurred in pregnancies terminating at less than 29 weeks and/or resulting in an infant whose birth weight was less than 1000 g. Five of the six women experiencing a loss had developed superimposed preeclampsia. Exacerbation of hypertension severe enough to require initiation of antihypertensive treatment occurred in 10.0% of the gravidas. Furthermore, 12.8% experienced hypertension accompanied by a minimum of 500 mg/day proteinuria. Seventeen (7.9%) of the newborns were small for gestational age (SGA). Almost half the women delivering SGA infants had developed superimposed preeclampsia. Twenty-six newborns (12.1%) were premature and 45 (20.9%) were less than 2500 g at birth. No benefit was felt to accrue from prophylactic treatment of mild hypertension.

Arias and Zamora treated 29 patients with mild diastolic hypertension (diastolic pressure less than 100 mm Hg) with combinations of methyldopa, hydralazine, and hydrochlorothiazide and compared maternal and neonatal outcome to a control group treated with no medications. They found that only 4/29 (13.8%) treated women vs 13/29 (44.8%) untreated women ($P < 0.05$) developed toxemia.[5] There were no differences in the average gestational age at birth, fetal weight, incidence of low Apgar scores, incidence of low-birth-weight infants, incidence of intrauterine growth retardation (IUGR), or fetal distress. One neonatal death occurred secondary to meconium aspiration (PMR = 17/1000). No attempt was made to differentiate between exacerbation of hypertension or development of preeclampsia. A reduced incidence of acute elevations of blood pressure or "pregnancy aggravated" hypertension justified treating with medication, although no benefit to the fetus could be documented.

A large, prospective, controlled, but not blinded, trial of antihypertensive therapy for the treatment of chronic hypertension in pregnancy was conducted by Redman et al.[6] Women noted, prior to the 28th gestational week, to have diastolic hypertension between 90 and 110 mm Hg were treated with alphamethyldopa. The difference in perinatal outcome in the study group, compared to women treated with no medication (Table 6-1) achieved statistical significance. Surprisingly, the improvement was due to a decrease in the

Table 6-1
Perinatal Mortality in Treated and Control Groups with Early Diagnosed Hypertension*

	Control		Treated		P
Enrolled in study	107		101		
Mid trimester stillborn	4		0		0.021
Late trimester stillborn	1	27 weeks, 700 g (AGA),† severe preeclampsia,	1	32 weeks, 1600 g (AGA), intrapartum demise	
Neonatal death	1	38 weeks, 3800 g (AGA), no preeclampsia, precipitate labor, death at 18 hours, intraventricular hemorrhage	0		
Survivors	101	(94.4%)	100	(99.0%)	0.021

*Redman CWG, Beilin LJ, Bunner J: Fetal outcome in trial of antihypertensive treatment in pregnancy. *Lancet* 1976;2:754.
†AGA = Appropriate for gestational age.

number of mid-trimester stillbirths that were unassociated with exacerbations of blood pressure.

The conflicting results summarized above both serve as the justification for using antihypertensive agents in the management of pregnancy complicated by chronic hypertension and as the justification for not treating patients with medication. The controversy has been further complicated by the recent introduction and acceptance by internists of a new class of antihypertensive agents, the beta blockers. The initial reluctance by obstetricians to the use of this group of drugs has diminished as more cardiospecific drugs in the same class have been developed. Evaluation of these newer drugs has shown them to be safer. However, far from settled, as yet, is proof of efficacy or advantage over older, well-known drugs.

The most common maternal complication of pregnancy already complicated by chronic hypertension is the acute exacerbation of hypertension, which is often followed by the need to prematurely terminate the pregnancy. Hauth et al evaluated the results of 372 young nulliparas with elevated blood pressures, admitted for prolonged sedentary hospitalization.[7] A normal diet without diuretics, sedatives, or antihypertensive agents was preserved. Frequent evaluations of blood pressure, weight, and proteinuria, were complemented by serial studies of renal function, coagulation, and fetal growth. Labor was induced upon maternal or fetal deterioration, inducibility near/at term, or spontaneous rupture of the membranes. Of the 346 patients who completed the in-hospital course of thereapy, 292/346 (84.4%) became normotensive within five days and 314/346 (90.8%) delivered at term after spending an average of 24 days in the hospital and experienced a PMR of 9/1000. Twenty-six patients left the hospital against medical advice after an average length of stay of 13 days; four fetal and no neonatal deaths occurred (PMR 154/1000). These impressive results of prompt recognition and in-hospital management of acute exacerbations of hypertension could not be expected to be duplicated in an older population suffering from chronic hypertension. However, as the acute complications that do befall the older hypertensive gravida are well known and not difficult to diagnose, they may be capable of similar modification, amelioration, and successful treatment.

DIABETES MELLITUS

Another common medical complication that impacts on the reproductive performance of the older gravida is diabetes mellitus. The Joslin Diabetes Clinic experience revealed immediate improvement in maternal survival and a more gradual improvement in perinatal survival associated with the discovery and introduction of insulin.[8] Maternal mortality decreased from 34% in 1898–1938 to 1% in 1938–1974; perinatal mortality decreased from 46% to 14% during this same period, dropped to 10% in 1958–1974, and further decreased to 6% in 1975. In 1975–1978, 147 women who attained 24 gestational weeks were managed by a team of obstetricians and internists stressing diet, weekly antenatal visits, frequent urine and infrequent blood analysis in attempting to achieve normoglycemia without incapacitating hypoglycemia.[9] Assessment of metabolic control, based on the standards of O'Sullivan et al,[10] revealed that most patients were far from normoglycemic. Perinatal mortality (Table 6-2) was lower than in previous decades, but morbidity was high. A subsequent report from the Joslin Clinic, evaluating 35 class F (nephropathy) patients, revealed a marked reduction in perinatal mortality, even in these very ill diabetic patients.[11]

Gabbe et al also attempted to achieve normoglycemia—a fasting blood glucose (FBG) of 100–110 mg/dl and a postprandial glucose (PPG) of less than 140 mg/dl.[12] Patients received in-hospital education, diet instruction, and insulin administration training followed by weekly outpatient visits. All patients were hospitalized at 34 weeks; delivery was based on individual evaluation of fetal lung maturity and/or maternal/fetal deterioration.

There were no maternal deaths; the stillbirth rate was the same as the nondiabetic population, but two thirds of the infants experienced some type of morbidity including congenital defects (7%), respiratory distress syndrome (6%), delivery trauma (3%), macrosomia (22%), and "frequent" episodes of hypoglycemia, hypocalcemia, and erythemia (Table 6-3). Perinatal mortality was not related to advanced maternal age.

Table 6-2
Perinatal Mortality and Morbidity in Infants of Diabetic Mothers*

White class	Number of patients	Number of stillbirths	Number of neonatal deaths	Congenital anomalies	Comments
A	13	0	0	0	
B	30	1	1	0	1 stillborn, maternal ketoacidosis, 1 neonatal death at 28 weeks, respiratory distress syndrome
C	57	0	0	6	
D	37	0	2	6	1 neonatal death, multiple malformations 1 neonatal death, respiratory distress syndrome at 30 weeks
F	8	0	1	1	1 neonatal death, abruption, intrapartum asphyxia
R	2	0	0	0	
Total	147	1	4	13	Perinatal mortality rate: 34/1000

*Kitzmiller JL, Brown ER, Phillipe M, et al: Diabetic nephropathy and perinatal outcome. *Am J Obstet Gynecol* 1981;141:741.

Table 6-3
Perinatal Mortality in Class B-R Diabetes*

White class	Number of patients	Number of stillborn	Number of neonatal deaths	Comment
B	190	2	6	1 stillborn, multiple malformations 1 stillborn, Rh disease
C	38	1	0	
D	23	0	2	2 neonatal deaths, multiple malformations
F	6	0	0	
R	3	0	0	
Total	260	3	8	Perinatal mortality rate: 42/1000

*Gabbe S, Mestman JH, Freeman RL: Management and outcome of pregnancy in diabetes mellitus, class B-R. *Am J Obstet Gynecol* 1973;129:723.

Table 6-4
Glucose Levels in Pregnant Diabetics

	Mean preprandial glucose (mg/dl) group*		
	<115	*115–172*	*>172*
Number of patients	18	79	24
Perinatal mortality	0	2†(25.3/1000)	3‡(125/1000)
Morbidity	Incidence within each group (%)		
Hypoglycemia	40	26	24
Hypocalcemia	17	10	24
Hyperbilirubinemia	11	19	19
Respiratory distress	0	8	14
Macrosomia	28	40	33
Malformations	0	9	17

*Loveno KJ, Hauth JC, Gilstrap LC: Appraisal of "rigid" blood glucose control during pregnancy in overtly diabetic women. *Am J Obstet Gynecol* 1979;135:853.

†1 trisomy 18, 1 cytomegaloviremia.

‡1 noncompliant patient, 1 congenital abnormality, 1 abruption.

Loveno et al evaluated pregnancy outcome in 121 women to assess if there was a relationship between degree of metabolic control and outcome.[13] The goal of metabolic management was <1+ glycosuria, a postprandial glucose <150 mg/dl, and a fasting blood glucose <115 mg/dl. Protocols for medical and obstetrical management were similar to those of Gabbe et al.[12]

Normoglycemia was felt to be both difficult to achieve and not without the risk of hypoglycemic episodes. Perinatal mortality was low in spite of "less than optimal control" and not related to maternal age (Table 6-4). Morbidity was high but, if control was poor, morbidity was not related to a worsening of already poor control.

Jovanovic et al evaluated the feasibility of maintaining optimal metabolic levels of glucose in an ambulatory setting in 10 women who were 21–32 years of age (average 27.5 years), less than eight weeks pregnant upon initiating the program, and overtly diabetic for 1–23 years (average 7).[14] A brief hospitalization (5–7 days) achieved a fasting plasma glucose of 60–70 mg/dl, a mean plasma glucose of 80–87 mg/dl, and a postprandial glucose of < 140 mg/dl. While in the hospital, the patients were offered nutritional education, division of their insulin regimen into three doses, and hourly glucose measurements. Following discharge, outpatient alterations of insulin dose and diet were based on at least five finger-sticks per day. Irrespective of glucose control, the patients were re-admitted at 20 and 36 weeks. After the first five days of the initial hospitalization, the group's mean glucose decreased from 169 mg/dl to 86 mg/dl, and all had normal glucose concentrations throughout their pregnancies. Hemoglobin Alc decreased to "normal" within five weeks. Hypoglycemic reactions (1/week) ceased after the first two weeks. The 10 women experienced a mean weight gain of 12.3 kg, and all delivered at 37–40 weeks (mean 39 weeks). Their babies weighed 2590–3200 g (mean 2988 g), had 5-minute Apgar scores of 10, and none experienced hypoglycemia, hypocalcemia, hyperbilirubinemia, erythemia, or respiratory distress syndrome.

A larger study, with a control diabetic population, was initiated. Initial outcomes in the control group included macrosomia, hypoglycemia, and shoulder dystocia; the control group was therefore abolished. The results in the enlarged study population included: (1) The preprogram mean glucose (202 mg/dl) and Hemoglobin Alc (120% of normal) were reduced to "normal" within one to two weeks. The mean glucose at delivery was 87 mg/dl. (2) No decrease in renal function or ocular status was noted. (3) Neither polyhydramnios nor urinary tract infections occurred. (4) There were no stillborns. (5) The mean delivery age for the entire group was 39 weeks. The mean delivery age for the white class D, R, and F subgroup was 37 weeks. (6) No infant's weight was greater than the 75th percentile or less than the 48th percentile, although infants of mothers with vascular involvement were lower in weight.[7] No major or minor congenital abnormalities were noted. No hypoglycemia, hypocalcemia, erythemia, hyperbilirubinemia, or respiratory distress syndrome occurred.[15] The authors concluded that the maintenance of euglycemia is both possible and not associated with significant risk, and may be a major determinant in the further reduction of perinatal mortality and morbidity.

Miller et al related the incidence of major malformations in infants of diabetic mothers to control of hyperglycemia in early pregnancy.[16] Prospective studies in Europe and the United States are currently underway attempting to diminish the incidence of birth defects by preconception or very early pregnancy strict metabolic control.

In the past, many fetuses of diabetic gravidas died abruptly in the last four weeks of the pregnancy or from complications of prematurity. Modern management protocols have markedly improved perinatal survival, although fetal and neonatal losses still occur in association with advanced diabetes or secondary to severe congenital malformations. Neonatal morbidity remains high; however if the work of Jovanovic can be duplicated by others, these complications may be brought under control.

ELDERLY GRAVIDA

The previously described Collaborative Perinatal Project (CPP) also provided data relating maternal age to pregnancy outcome.[17] Included in the total population studied were 2590 women between 35 and 39 years of age, 756 women who were greater than 39 years of age, and a total of 1435 autopsy reports on all infants who died between 20 weeks of gestation and 28 days after birth. Stillbirths accounted for 92% of the increased perinatal mortality that was associated with maternal age (Table 6-5). The perinatal mortality in pregnancies complicated by diabetes was so increased in both the young and the older gravidas that any possible additional con-

Table 6-5
Relationship of Maternal Age and Perinatal Mortality*

	Mother's age			
	20–30	*35–39*	*>39*	*P*†
Stillbirths/1000				
Black	18	30	53	<0.001
White	12	26	49	<0.001
Neonatal deaths	14	17	18	>0.1
Diabetes mellitus				
Absent	14	26	49	<0.001
Present	68	121	163	>0.1
Hypertension				
Absent	13	23	37	<0.001
Present	27	45	97	<0.005

**P* compares patients aged 20–30 to those >35 years of age.
†Naeye RL: Maternal age, obstetric complications, and the outcome of pregnancy. *Obstet Gynecol* 1983;61:210.

tribution of advancing maternal age could not be detected. The PMR of pregnancies complicated by hypertension was further worsened by advancing maternal age.

Birth order, paternal age, and maternal age were correlated to pregnancy outcome during the same decade as the CPP study in a review of 471,846 birth and fetal death certificates of white, singleton, newborns recorded in New York State.[18] Results (Table 6-6) reveal that paternal age and birth order, in addition to maternal age, contribute significantly and equally to the risk of fetal death.

Horger and Smythe compared the outcome of 440 pregnancies in women over age 40 (among 27,185 deliveries at the Medical University of South Carolina) during the years 1965–1974 to a control group of 1517 patients selected at random.[19] Study and control groups were composed of black women of low socioeconomic status. The perinatal mortality of the pregnancies in the 345 pregnancies that terminated in the birth of an infant weighing more than 500 g was 101/1000

Table 6-6
Relationship between Birth Order, Paternal and Maternal Age, and Fetal Loss*

	Fetal loss/1000 pregnancies
Birth order	
1	12.1
4	14.2
6+	23.5
Paternal age (years)	
20–25	9.7
35–39	16.7
45–49	28.9
>55	32.2
Maternal age (years)	
20–24	9.4
35–39	21.5
40–44	32.2
>45	51.3

*Selvin S, Garfinkel J: Paternal age, maternal age and birth order and the risk of a fetal loss. *Hum Biol* 1976;48:223.

(Table 6-7). This was more than triple the PMR in the hospital and was, as also noted in the Collaborative Perinatal Project, largely the result of stillbirths. The rate was also twice that seen in the Collaborative Perinatal Project, suggesting the contributing influence of poverty. Neonatal morbidity (defined as an Apgar score of ≤6, the need for respiratory assistance, or evidence of central nervous system problems) occurred in 48 (15.3%) of 314 live-born infants. Neonatal deaths occurred in 4 (8.3%) and congenital abnormalities occurred in 12 (25.0%) of these 48 infants. Three of the 31 (9.6%) fetal deaths and one of the four neonatal deaths were associated with the congenital defects.

Hypertensive vascular disease with or without superimposed preeclampsia was present in 120 (34.7%) patients. Isolated preeclampsia was diagnosed in 32 (9.3%) patients. Together these 152 patients accounted for 70.0% of the still-

Table 6-7
Reproductive Outcome of Older Gravida*

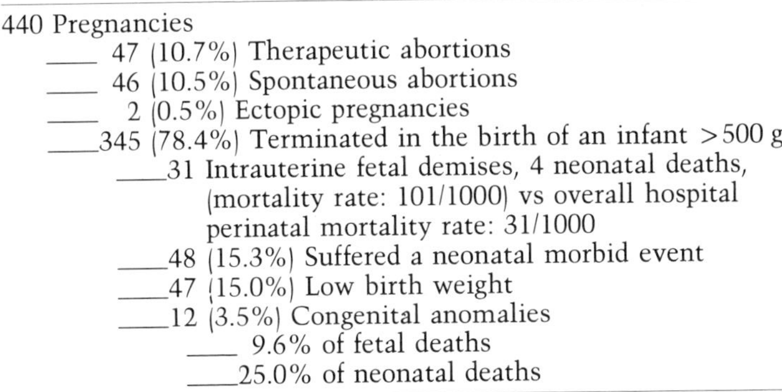

440 Pregnancies
- 47 (10.7%) Therapeutic abortions
- 46 (10.5%) Spontaneous abortions
- 2 (0.5%) Ectopic pregnancies
- 345 (78.4%) Terminated in the birth of an infant >500 g
  - 31 Intrauterine fetal demises, 4 neonatal deaths, (mortality rate: 101/1000) vs overall hospital perinatal mortality rate: 31/1000
  - 48 (15.3%) Suffered a neonatal morbid event
  - 47 (15.0%) Low birth weight
  - 12 (3.5%) Congenital anomalies
    - 9.6% of fetal deaths
    - 25.0% of neonatal deaths

*Horger EO, Smythe AR: Pregnancy in women over forty. *Obstet Gynecol* 1975;121:465.

borns and 75.0% of the neonatal deaths. Thirty-two patients 9.3%) were known to be diabetic or had abnormal glucose tolerance test during pregnancy or immediately postpartum. These 32 patients accounted for 19.4% of the stillborns and 50.0% of the neonatal deaths.

Kajanoja and Widholm described the reproductive outcome of 558 Finnish women aged 40 or greater who delivered 564 infants during 1969–1975 at Helsinki University Central Hospital.[20] Morbidity for the gravidas was high. Maternal intrahepatic cholestasis, a disorder common among Scandinavian women, occurred in 3% of women; hypertension occurred in 31%; the incidence of diabetes and rhesus incompatibility were high partly due to the centralization of high-risk gravida to this hospital. In spite of high morbidity, no severe deterioration in maternal health or maternal death occurred.

The average duration of labor was six hours; in only six patients did labor last longer than 18 hours. The incidence of cesarean section for primiparas was 31% (almost three times that for the general population); the rate for multiparas was 21%.

The PMR of 28/1000 for this homogeneous white population should be compared to the aforementioned rate for low socioeconomic black women (101/1000), emphasizing the difficulty in ascertaining the real PMR of the older gravida and the confounding element of poverty to reproductive outcome. As expected, 13 of the 16 (81.3%) deaths were fetal; there were no intrapartum fetal deaths. Of the 13 stillbirths, nine (69.2%) weighed less than 2500 g; eleven (84.6%) were caused by anoxia associated with placental infarcts, abruption, or insufficiency; one stillbirth resulted from a cord accident, and one resulted from multiple malformations. The prematurity rate was higher than for the general population (12% vs 6%), and the incidence of small-for-gestational-age neonates was 9% (data for general population unavailable). The three neonatal deaths were the result of immaturity (700 g), respiratory distress in a 1740-g infant, and erythroblastosis in a 1880-g infant. Data was not available to compare the 5.6% congenital abnormality rate discovered at birth to the rate in the general population; Down's syndrome represented 40.6% of the discovered defects.

Morrison reviewed the pregnancy outcome of 127 primigravidas (0.64% of the obstetric population), aged 35 years or older who delivered in Winnipeg, Canada, during 1968–1972.[21] The oldest woman was 46 years old. The control group consisted of a random selection of primigravidas less than 35 years of age. Infant follow-up continued for five years.

The uncorrected PMR of this study group was 94/1000 (similar to Horger and Smythe) and consisted of six stillbirths and six neonatal deaths. Corrected for congenital abnormalities incompatible with life and for infants with birth weights less than 1000 g, PMR was reduced to 47/1000. The incidence of neonatal morbid events (defined similarly to

Horger and Smythe) and number of small-for-gestational-age infants was increased. The difference in the prematurity rate for the study group (14%) and the control group (5%) did not reach statistical significance. Pregnancies of duration greater than 40 weeks associated with labors lasting greater than 20 hours contributed 75% of the infants who suffered morbid events. The incidence of congenital abnormalities was 3%, which did not differ significantly from the general population.

Blum, during the same decade, evaluated 57 primiparas, mostly aged 35–38 years, representing 0.65% of all primiparas delivering in the Hasharion Hospital, Israel.[22] Control groups consisted of 97 primiparas aged 30–34 years of age and another group of 250 primiparas between 20 and 29 years of age. The incidence of preeclampsia, hypertension, diabetes, low Apgar scores, and the PMR (36/1000 live births) was similar for the three groups, although the incidence of SGA babies (14.5%) was greater in the study group compared to youngest gravidas. A striking difference in the cesarean section rate (49%) as compared to 2.3% in the group aged 20–29 years of age, makes outcomes difficult to analyze and points to a solution to (or the creation of another problem) the poor perinatal performance of the older gravida.

Hay and Barbano abstracted data from birth certificates of white singleton deliveries from 29 states during 1961–1966 to evaluate the relationship between maternal age, birth order, and the incidence of congenital malformations (Table 6-8).[23] Most malformations are underreported on birth certificates; however, underreporting should not be biased in relation to maternal age or birth order. The most dramatic trend was the positive association of Down's syndrome with increasing maternal age in every category of birth order. (The data did not reveal an excess of first births, in any maternal age groups, resulting in Down's syndrome.) Congenital heart defects also showed a positive trend with maternal age but to a lesser degree and with less consistency; this trend persisted

Table 6-8
Incidence of Birth Defects*

Congenital defect	Maternal Age	
	20–24	*40+*
	Defects/100,000 births	
I. Nervous system		
1. Anencephaly	26	24
2. Spina bifida	70	86
3. Hydrocephaly	34	39
II. Cardiovascular		
1. Congenital heart disease	60	129
III. Chromosomal		
1. Down's syndrome	22	559
IV. Facial		
1. Cleft lip and palate	52	89
2. Cleft lip without cleft palate	32	30
3. Cleft palate without cleft lip	37	58
V. Gastrointestinal		
1. Tracheoesophageal fistula, other esophageal defects	11	16
2. Omphalocele	18	19
VI. Genitourinary		
1. Imperforate anus, other anorectal disorders	23	38
2. Hypospadias	66	65
VII. Orthopedic		
1. Positional foot defects	140	166
2. Polydactyly	48	60
3. Syndactyly	24	35
4. Reduction deformities	31	42

*Hay S, Barbano H: Independent effects of maternal age and birth order on the incidence of selected congenital abnormalities. *Teratology* 1972;6:271.

even when children with Down's syndrome with congenital heart disease were excluded. Although the majority of defects revealed at least some relationship to advancing age, a significant increase in rates was not noted until the oldest maternal age groups were reached.

CONCLUSIONS

Improvement in reproductive outcome for all gravidas has resulted from both social and medical advances. The availability of liberal contraceptive, abortion, and sterilization services in association with technological and philosophical advances in obstetrical and neonatal care have led to improved perinatal survival rates, diminished perinatal morbidity, and improved maternal outcome. In the face of an overall improved reproductive outcome, what specifically can be proposed to the older woman to help her and her family wisely choose the best reproductive course?

Prepregnancy counseling that includes a discussion of both the risks and benefits of contraceptive techniques (temporary and permanent) should continue to be made available. Local, inexpensive, and free-of-bureaucratic-hassle access to unbiased reproductive counselors will permit each woman to choose the initiation, termination, or continuation of her pregnancy according to her needs.

All women over aged 35 should be offered prepregnancy or early pregnancy birth defects counseling services and information. Irrespective of the health care provider's attitude towards amniocentesis and/or abortion, there is a medical and legal responsibility to inform patients of the risks and significance of delivery and/or aborting a fetus with Down's syndrome. Screening for open spinal defects using serum alpha-fetoprotein is both technically feasible and, especially for the older gravida, a cost-effective measure. Although additional congenital defects may, in the future, be detected by early pregnancy chemical or ultrasound evaluation, no other population-wide screening test is currently available.

Various protocols for diabetic screening and management have been described. The cost effectiveness for the general population and the clinical validity of random, fasting, or 1 or 2 hour postprandial glucose determinations following either a glucose challenge or a high carbohydrate breakfast remain controversial. However, the increasing incidence of diabetes in the older population and the demonstrated decrease in morbidity and mortality for the recognized and well-controlled diabetic gravida make a compelling argument for screening, in some way, women or gravidas over the age of 35. Prepregnancy glucose screening offers the opportunity to diagnose and treat hyperglycemia prior to conception and possibly prevent hyperglycemia related birth defects. Early pregnancy screening will allow diagnosis of diabetes and time to permit evaluation for diagnosable congenital defects and to reduce fetal morbidity and mortality.

Prepregnancy or early pregnancy evaluation for hypertension is a common clinical activity. Availability of health care providers, either physician, nurse, or trained paraprofessional, to evaluate blood pressure is or should be a continuing public health care priority. Undiagnosed and untreated hypertension in a 35-year-old woman or gravida should and can be eliminated.

Increasing the public's awareness of the necessity for early pregnancy prenatal visits should continue to be a priority for local public health agencies. This will allow the primary health care provider to assess the combined effects of age, gravidity, social situation, and coexisting medical illnesses. Awareness of medical conditions, most often hypertension or diabetes, in association with pregnancy mandates a combined medical–obstetrical team approach to pregnancy management. Frequent consultation among physicians, frequent prenatal visits, cessation of stressful activities (including work, if necessary), and frequent and often prolonged hospitalization may be necessary to ensure the optimum outcome. Early planning and mobilization of resources for referral and delivery in tertiary-care facilities must include family members, health care providers, public health nurses, and social workers to ensure minimum disruption in family life and maximum chances for a good outcome for mother and baby.

REFERENCES

1. Adams MM, Oakley GP, Marks JS: Maternal age and births in the 1980's. *JAMA* 1982;247:493.
2. Friedman EA, Neff R: Hypertension-hypotension in pregnancy. *JAMA* 1978;239:2249.
3. Naeye R, Friedman EA: Causes of death associated with gestational hypertension and proteinuria. *Am J Obstet Gynecol* 1978;133:8.
4. Sabii BM, Abdella TN, Anderson GD: Pregnancy outcome in 211 patients with mild hypertension. *Obstet Gynecol* 1983;61:571.
5. Arias F, Zamora J: Anti-hypertensive treatment and pregnancy outcome in patients with mild hypertension. *Obstet Gynecol* 1979;53:489.
6. Redman CWG, Beilin LJ, Bunner J: Fetal outcome in trial of antihypertensive treatment in pregnancy. *Lancet* 1976;2:754.
7. Hauth JC, Cunningham FG, Walley P: Management of pregnancy induced hypertension in the nullipara. *Obstet Gynecol* 1976; 48:253.
8. Hare JW, White P: Pregnancy in diabetes complicated by vascular disease. *Diabetes* 1977;26:953.
9. Kitzmiller J, Cloherty JP, Younger DM, et al: Diabetic pregnancy and perinatal morbidity. *Am J Obstet Gynecol* 1978;131:560.
10. O'Sullivan JB, Mahan CM, Charles D: Medical treatment of the gestational diabetic. *Obstet Gynecol* 1974;43:817.
11. Kitzmiller JL, Brown ER, Phillippe M, et al: Diabetic nephropathy and perinatal outcome. *Am J Obstet Gynecol* 1981;141:741.
12. Gabbe S, Mestman JH, Freeman RK: Management and outcome of pregnancy in diabetes mellitus, class B-R. *Am J Obstet Gynecol* 1973;129:723.
13. Loveno KJ, Hauth JC, Gilstrap LC: Appraisal of "rigid" blood glucose control during pregnancy in overtly diabetic women. *Am J Obstet Gynecol* 1979;135:853.
14. Jovanovic L, Peterson CM, Saxena BB: Feasibility of maintaining normal glucose profiles in insulin dependent pregnant diabetic women. *Am J Med* 1980;68:105–111.
15. Jovanovic L, Druzin M, Peterson CM: Effect of euglycemia on the outcome of pregnancy in insulin dependent diabetic women as compared to normal controls. *Am J Med* 1981;71:521.
16. Miller E, Hare JW, Cloherty JP, et al: Elevated maternal hemoglobin Alc in early pregnancy and major congenital anomalies in infants of diabetic mothers. *N Engl J Med* 1981;304:1331.

17. Naeye RL: Maternal age, obstetric complications, and the outcome of pregnancy. *Obstet Gynecol* 1983;61:210.
18. Selvin S, Garfinkel J: Paternal age, maternal age and birth order and the risk of a fetal loss. *Hum Biol* 1976;48:223.
19. Horger EO, Smythe AR: Pregnancy in women over forty. *Obstet Gynecol* 1975;121:465.
20. Kajanoja P, Widholm O: Pregnancy and delivery in women aged 40 and over. *Obstet Gynecol* 1978;51:47.
21. Morrison I: The elderly primigravida. *Am J Obstet Gynecol* 1975;121:465.
22. Blum M: Is the elderly primipara really at high risk. *Medicine (Baltimore)* 1979;7:108.
23. Hay S, Barbano H: Independent effects of maternal age and birth order on the incidence of selected congenital abnormalities. *Teratology* 1972;6:271.

CHAPTER 7

CONGENITAL MALFORMATIONS: EPIDEMIOLOGY, DETECTION, AND PREVENTION

Barbara R. Pober, MD
L.B. Holmes, MD

In Western countries, congenital malformations are a leading cause of perinatal morbidity and mortality. As infant mortality from all causes has steadily declined in the United States, the portion of mortality attributable to congenital malformations has continued to increase. Approximately 21% of infant deaths were due to congenital malformations in 1981.[1] This finding, in combination with the trend toward diminished family size, has fostered intense public and professional interest in means of reducing the prevalence of malformed newborns.

This chapter will describe: (1) the prevalence of several types of major malformations occurring in different populations and geographic regions, (2) the methods available to diagnose prenatally the presence of a malformed fetus, and (3) the methods available to prevent or diminish the likelihood of developing a malformed fetus. This chapter will also consider the public health impact that both prevention and prenatal diagnosis have on reducing the prevalence of malformed newborns.

DEFINITION OF CONGENITAL MALFORMATIONS

Congenital malformations are generally defined as "structural malformations of prenatal origin."[2] Unfortunately, there are no universal standards for what constitutes a malformation and diagnoses are subject to individual (observer) bias. Many investigators have attempted to restrict the definition of the structural defects to those that alter the life of the affected individual (ie, a defect that requires some medical or surgical attention).[3,4] Infants born with anencephaly or omphalocele unequivocably have a major congenital malformation; it is far less clear whether cases affected with either a metabolic disturbance such as phenylketonuria, or malformations of lesser impact such as polydactyly or hydrocele should be similarly classified. Many investigators devise unique definitions, and, as a result, the number of so-called major malformations ascertained in a given study can vary widely. This lack of standardization poses particular problems for interstudy comparisons.

Minor malformations are generally considered to be those "abnormalities" occurring in less than 4% of infants which do not alter or compromise the affected individual's life.[5] Again, there are no universal standards or definitions for the diagnosis of minor malformations. However, their isolated presence has such limited public health importance that the remainder of the discussion will focus only on major malformations.

ETIOLOGIC CLASSIFICATION

Despite variation as to what should be considered a malformation, the spectrum of human birth defects can be categorized into groups of presumed or apparent etiology (Table 7-1). Malformations secondary to multifactorial inheritance comprise 20–30% of known etiologies, while

Table 7-1
Malformations by Apparent Etiology

Apparent etiology	Examples	Percent of all malformations		
		Holmes et al[3]	*Kalter and Warkany*[2]	*Fraser*[6]
Genetic abnormalities				
Chromosome abnormalities	Trisomy 21	6.6	6.0	10
Single gene abnormalities	Meckel-Gruber syndrome	3.0	7.5	5
Familial, but pattern of inheritance uncertain	Polydactyly	18.0*	—†	—
Multifactorial inheritance	Neural tube defects, cleft lip and cleft palate	31.2	20	20
Environmental factors		4.0	5	5
Maternal conditions	Diabetes mellitus, intrauterine infections	3.8	—	—
Teratogenic drugs	Phenytoin, chemotherapy	1.2	—	—
Environmental exposures	Ionizing radiation	—	—	—
Unknown cause	Diaphragmatic hernia, gastroschisis	30.7	60	60

*This category apparently included in "unknown cause" by references 2 and 6.
†Information not available.

chromosomal anomalies comprise 6–10%, monogenic abnormalities 3–7.5%, and environmental factors 4–5%.[2,3,6] Unfortunately, 50–60% of all malformed infants cannot be placed in an etiologic category at the present time. The remaining small percentages of malformed infants are divided among the other categories depicted in Table 7-1.

Estimates of relative frequency of malformations are complicated. The actual percentages differ according to the population studied and the methods used for ascertainment and diagnosis. The frequency of chromosomal anomalies will serve as a case in point. The prevalence of all chromosomal anomalies (detected by banding techniques) among consecutively karyotyped live-borns is approximately 0.6–0.7%[7,8] whereas the prevalence in a population of live-born and stillborn infants karyotyped solely on the basis of malformations and/or dysmorphic appearance is 0.16%.[3] However, the prevalence among a population of fetuses karyotyped at 16 weeks of gestation during amniocentesis is 2.3%.[9] These differences reflect underascertainment based on clinical criteria, the higher frequency of chromosomal anomalies among fetuses versus term infants, and the differing maternal age distributions of these groups.

EPIDEMIOLOGY OF MAJOR MALFORMATIONS

Descriptive epidemiologic studies of major malformation prevalence rates have been performed throughout the world. These studies provide information to help determine local environmental and genetic causes of malformations. If "preventable" factors can be identified, then intervention may decrease the occurrence of a given anomaly. Interstudy comparisons can be complicated since observed differences in prevalence rates may not be attributable to underlying population or environmental differences, but rather to differences

Table 7-2
Difficulties Making Interstudy Comparisons

Methodologic differences	Demographic differences
Definition of malformation	Racial composition
Diagnosis of malformation (direct exam, medical record, vital statistics)	Age composition
Ascertainment of live births vs live births and stillbirths	Socioeconomic composition
Variable length of follow-up	Geographic distribution
Inclusion of multiple births	Calendar time
Inclusion of malformed siblings	
Tabulation of multiple malformations/infant	
Maternal transfer status (for hospital-based study)	
Ascertainment and inclusion of malformed spontaneous abortuses	

in study design and definitions. Study differences fall into two broad categories (Table 7-2).

Examples of selected prevalence rates are presented (Appendix 7-1).[4,10–19] Methodologic differences, such as length of follow-up, strongly affect the observed prevalence rate. This variable alone can explain the almost fourfold higher major malformation rate found in the Collaborative Perinatal Project (which ascertained up to 1 year of age) compared to studies restricting ascertainment to the newborn period.[4,11,15,16] However, true population differences appear to exist as well. For example, studies performing actual physical examinations demonstrate the prevalence rate of polydactyly to be eightfold higher among Ugandan blacks compared to American whites.[4,12] The rates of cleft lip and cleft palate show a general pattern of a two- or threefold elevation among

Oriental infants (both Japanese and Chinese) compared to Caucasians and blacks.[10,12–16] These studies suggest there are varying genetic predispositions to specific defects, but contributory environmental factors cannot be ruled out.

Another example of population differences is variation in occurrence of neural tube defects (NTDs). Prevalence rates for Western European Caucasians, particularly those from Northern Ireland and northwest Great Britain, are consistently higher than for other Caucasian, Oriental, and black populations.[20–22] However, even within seemingly homogeneous Caucasian populations, such as within the United Kingdom, prevalence rates within a single geographic region have varied over time. Circumscribed "epidemics" or "clusters" are well documented.[20,23,24] Finally, there has been a recent decline in NTD prevalence rates beyond what is attributable to elective pregnancy terminations.[25–27] This suggests that both genetic and environmental factors play a significant contributory role in the development of NTDs. These findings have prompted more "in-depth" studies that attempt to identify causal and preventable factors[20,28–30] which, in turn may be used to control or prevent the development of NTDs.

PRENATAL DETECTION OF MAJOR MALFORMATIONS

There are a number of diagnostic techniques now available that can detect the presence of fetal malformations. Several of these are implemented via mass screening programs (such as maternal serum alpha-fetoprotein screening) whereas others are restricted toward high-risk pregnancies (such as fetal tissue sampling). The effectiveness of these methodologies depends on: (1) in utero detection and diagnosis of malformations after they have developed and (2) elective termination of affected pregnancies. Specific methodologies will first be highlighted followed by evaluation of some existing and proposed screening programs.

Chorionic Villus Biopsy

First trimester transcervical biopsy of the zygote-derived chorionic villus has been successfully used for purposes of prenatal diagnosis.[31] The collection of villus samples permits direct chromosomal analysis,[32] fetal sex determination,[33,34] restriction endonuclease analysis of DNA,[35] and enzyme analysis.[36] The expanding repertoire of gene-specific and chromosome-specific probes will increase the diagnostic capabilities of this technique in the future.

The impetus behind this technique has been that the procedure can be performed in the first trimester, the diagnosis can generally be established within hours to days, and an earlier diagnosis permits easier and potentially safer pregnancy termination. On the other hand, the safety of the procedure has not been thoroughly and systematically evaluated. The estimate of a 5% spontaneous abortion rate following the procedure may be excessively high,[31,37] but newer data is not available. A recent estimate of a 1% fetal loss rate among control pregnancies at a similar gestational age suggests there indeed may be some excess risk attributable to the procedure.[38] The magnitude of this risk may fall with improved technology and operator experience.

The procedure has been restricted to pregnancies known to be at high risk for diagnosable genetic, chromosomal, or biochemical disorders (eg, where the risk of the disorder is greater than the presumed risk of the procedure).[37] Under such circumstances, the public health impact of chorionic villus sampling is limited. Future impact could be greater as the diagnostic capabilities increase and as the risks of the procedure are better defined so that it may be used in other (lower risk) indications.

AMNIOCENTESIS

Midtrimester withdrawal of amniotic fluid is now routinely accepted for prenatal diagnosis of a variety of chromosomal abnormalities, genetic disorders, and even one class of multifactorial disorders—neural tube defects. The procedure involves transabdominal aspiration of amniotic fluid from the amniotic sac under ultrasound guidance at approximately 16 weeks' gestation.[39] The safety of this procedure has been prospectively evaluated in three multicenter clinical trials.[40–42] Despite study design differences (primarily that of finding an appropriate comparison group), the collective data show that in the hands of an experienced operator, using a small gauge needle and not requiring repeated "taps," amniocentesis is a safe procedure with low risks to the mother and the fetus. A demonstrable, although not significant statistically, excess fetal loss rate (including spontaneous abortions, stillbirths, and perinatal deaths) of approximately 1% was reported to occur in the amniocentesis group.[40,41] Since these reports, ultrasound guidance at the time of the procedure is routine so that most recent estimates of postprocedure loss are lower than 1.0%.[39,42] Some of the small excess appears attributable to the procedure itself and some to the nature of the high-risk pregnancy undergoing the procedure. Other reported complications in the past have included an increased frequency of musculoskeletal anomalies[41] (subsequently unsubstantiated),[43] increased neonatal respiratory distress,[41] rare case reports of fetal puncture,[44] limb defects secondary to amniotic band constriction resulting from amnion puncture,[45] and fetal death secondary to needle puncture.[45a]

The sample of amniotic fluid collected during the procedure can be divided and used for different diagnostic purposes, depending on the original indication for the procedure.

Tests on amniotic fluid cells

Chromosome analysis Excellent quality preparations for chromosome analysis can be performed on cultured amniotic fluid cells.[46,47] The diagnostic accuracy of such analyses is high—approximately 99%.[40,42,48] Technical failures, results of unusual or questionable significance (such as low-level mosaicism or apparent translocation), errors in sex determination, and actual misdiagnoses are rare.[49]

Inherited metabolic disorders An increasing number of inherited metabolic disorders can now be diagnosed antenatally. Analysis for specific enzyme defects (or metabolic products secondary to such defects) in cultured amniotic fluid cells can be used to detect fetuses affected with sphingolipid, mucopolysaccharide, carbohydrate, amino acid, and other types of metabolic disorders.[50,51]

Recombinant DNA technology The recently developed recombinant DNA technology allows for identification of normal and abnormal gene sequences. In turn, this knowledge can be used for purposes of prenatal diagnosis. For example, the restriction enzyme MstII fortuitously cleaves the B-globin gene at the base sequence altered in sickle hemoglobin. Thus, it will produce different-sized DNA fragments in cells with the sickle mutation than in cells with the normal gene.[52,53] The presence of mutant genes can also be identified by the fortuitous linkage of the abnormal gene to "polymorphic" restriction sites. For example, there are multiple polymorphic restriction sites flanking the B-globin gene. Thus, within a given family, the linkage of certain sites to the mutant gene can be used to diagnose prenatally many forms of B-thalassemia.[53,54] DNA polymorphisms can also be used for the prenatal diagnosis of phenylketonuria,[55] and potentially for Huntington's disease.[56]

Use of closely linked genes This method is based on the linkage of mutant genes to identifiable polymorphic protein products. The prenatal diagnosis of 21-hydroxylase deficiency congenital adrenal hyperplasia has been made on the basis of the genetic linkage of the 21-hydroxylase gene and polymorphic HLA gene products.[57,58]

Tests on amniotic fluid Biochemical analysis on amniotic fluid has been directed primarily toward the prenatal diagnosis of neural tube defects (NTDs). The most widely used marker is alpha-fetoprotein (AFP), a major fetal protein first produced by the yolk sac and then the liver.[59] The peak concentration of AFP occurs in fetal blood at approximately 12 weeks of gestation and declines steadily thereafter.[60] During the second trimester, the concentration of AFP in fetal serum is normally 100–200 times higher than in amniotic fluid.[61,62] This normal ratio can be altered by a malformation, such as anencephaly or omphalocele, which permits leakage or transudation of fetal serum AFP directly into amniotic fluid.[61]

Elevated AFP and NTDs Normal and abnormal amniotic fluid AFP (AFAFP) levels have been established for specific gestational ages.[63] The data suggest that determination of AFAFP levels at the correct gestational age, and by an experienced and quality-controlled laboratory, can detect 98% of all cases of anencephaly and open spina bifida.[63,64] The accuracy of this test is therefore high, with a detection rate or sensitivity of 98% and a reported specificity of 99.5%.[63] Complete detection of affected cases does not seem possible, on the basis of AFAFP alone, due to a small amount of overlap between the range of "normal" AFAFP values and the "abnormal" values associated with open spina bifida.[65] Thus, if one lowers the cutoff level to enhance the detection rate, the false-positive rate will simultaneously increase.

There are many causes of an elevated AFAFP other than open neural tube defects (Table 7-3). Although the reason or reasons for elevated AFAFP usually become apparent, there remains justifiable concern that a small number of normal fetuses will be aborted because of an elevated AFAFP. The rate of false positives among normal singleton fetuses is

Table 7-3
Causes of Elevated AFAFP*
(other than NTDs)

Diagnosis	Management
1. Subsequent fetal loss[60,63,66]	None available
2. Underestimate of gestational age[67]	Improved gestational age dating by ultrasound examination
3. Fetal malformations such as omphalocoele, gastroschisis, congenital nephrosis (reviewed in 67)	Additional diagnostic work-up (eg, ultrasound study)
4. Blood-stained amniotic fluid[60,63]	Evaluate amniotic fluid for fetal blood;[61] repeat amniocentesis;[61] adjunct use of acetylcholinesterase[62]
5. Normal fetus (false positive result)[63]	

*Amniotic fluid alpha-fetoprotein.

generally reported to be between 0.1% and 0.5%.[63,67,68] Fortunately, the actual rate of termination of such fetuses is considerably lower (less than 0.1%) due to repeat and ancillary tests to confirm the presence of the presumed defect.[27,60,63]

False-negative AFAFP levels (levels below the cutoff value) occur in the presence of (1) closed NTDs such as skin-covered or membrane-covered meningoceles or encephaloceles[69]; (2) erroneously sampled maternal urine rather than amniotic fluid[60,70]; and (3) a few cases of open spina bifida.[63]

Acetylcholinesterase Acetylcholinesterase (ACHE) is one of a group of enzymes which hydrolyze choline esters found in high concentrations in brain, spinal cord, and serum.[61] Elevated amounts of amniotic fluid ACHE in the presence of an open NTD reflects direct leakage into the amniotic fluid[68,71] and over 99% of open NTDs result in elevated ACHE levels.[72] Blood contamination may also elevate amniotic fluid ACHE.[60,72] Adverse outcomes other than NTDs do not elevate amniotic fluid ACHE as consistently as they do AFAFP, and therefore this test has a more limited diagnostic range.[72]

Alkaline phosphatase Certain amniotic fluid analyses have been performed in the hope of prenatally diagnosing cystic fibrosis.[73,74,74a] The only potentially successful assay to date shows that low levels of an amniotic fluid alkaline phosphatase isoenzyme (a phenylalanine-inhibitable isoenzyme) can detect fetuses affected with cystic fibrosis.[73] Further details on the sensitivity and specificity of this test are currently lacking.

Two to three percent of pregnant women intending to carry to term currently undergo amniocentesis in England and Wales.[75] The utilization rate in the New England region of the United States was approximately 4% of all pregnancies in 1984.[76]

Data from several centers show similar reasons why amniocenteses were performed (Table 7-4). The most common indications for amniocentesis were a positive family history of some type of disorder or defect and advanced maternal age.[40,48,77] The relative proportion of each indication reflected local prevalence of given disorders, existence of certain screening programs, and availability of services.

Amniocentesis, as it is currently utilized, will impart only a small reduction in the prevalence of newborn infants with major malformations. Several factors contribute to this limitation. First, most screening programs directed toward diagnosing chromosomal anomalies (generally trisomy 21) are offered to women aged 35 and over. Women of this age group produce approximately 5% of all live births and approximately 20–25% of all infants with trisomy 21.[78,79] Thus, 75–80% of trisomy 21 births (and probably a similar proportion of other less frequently occurring aneuploid conditions) are occurring in women less than 35 years of age who are not routinely offered amniocentesis. The second major factor is the low rate of utilization. Twenty-five to 65% of infants with

Table 7-4
Indications for Amniocentesis

Indication	Percent of amniocenteses		
	Galjaard[77]	*NICHD*[40]	*Golbus et al*[48]
Maternal age >35 years	37	47	80
Family history of cytogenic disorder	17	32.6	8.6
Parental cytogenetic disorder	3.0	2.0	0.5
Miscellaneous cytogenetic disorder	11.6	7.8	1.8
Sex determination (for X-linked disorder)	4.6	2.0	1.6
Family history metabolic disorder	3.4	8.8	3.2
Family history of NTD (AFP determination)	23	—	4.0
Total	100%	100%	100%

Down's syndrome are born to women over the age of 35 who did not utilize the option of prenatal diagnosis (although utilization rates continue to rise).[49,76,80]

Methods to identify a higher proportion of chromosomally abnormal fetuses throughout the entire maternal age spectrum are being sought. These included maternal serum alpha-fetoprotein screening and, potentially, chromosomal analysis for the "double nucleolar organizing region" (dNOR) chromosome variant. It has been reported that a parent with a double nucleolar organizing region produces 47 XY + 21 or 47 XX + 21 offspring 20 times as often as a parent without this chromosome variant.[83] The biologic mechanism underlying this finding and the feasibility of implementing it into a screening test are unknown.

Cost–benefit analyses have evaluated amniocentesis programs based on advanced maternal age (either 35 or 40 years of age).[79,81,82] They have all projected varying amounts of economic savings (exact amounts depend on maternal age cutoff, consideration of "replacement" costs of an affected individual by a normal individual, etc).

As shown in Table 7-4, most other amniocenteses are performed because of a positive family history. However, the majority of all incident cases of genetic disorders (both monogenic and chromosomal), as well as NTDs, occur in the absence of a positive family history. For example, 90% of NTDs occur in the so-called "low-risk" family.[69] Thus, focusing services on previously affected families is of great benefit to them but has limited public health impact.

Even if it were possible to diagnose every chromosomal and monogenic disorder plus all NTDs (as well as the other rare disorders that cause elevated AFAFP) in every fetus, amniotic fluid analysis would currently make a prenatal diagnosis in only 16–21% of malformed infants (Table 7-1).

Fetoscopy and Fetal Tissue Sampling

Direct sampling of selected fetal tissues can be carried out during the second trimester of pregnancy.[84] Fetal blood is most reliably and safely obtained by puncture of umbilical vessels.[85] This technique is used primarily for the prenatal diagnosis of hemoglobinopathies (although many of these diagnoses can now be made by recombinant DNA technology on cultured amniotic fluid cells).[86] Other indications for fetal sampling have been the diagnosis of hemophilia, alpha$_1$-antitrypsin deficiency, immunodeficiency disorders, and evaluation of fetal hydrops.[84–86] Skin biopsy has been used for diagnosis of severe hereditary skin disorders[87] and liver biopsy for certain metabolic disorders not diagnosable on amniotic fluid cells.[88]

Maternal risks from the procedure are negligible, and the reported risk of immediate and delayed fetal loss is between 1.0 and 5.0%,[86,89] suggesting that there is a small excess risk of loss attributable to the procedure.

Fetoscopy has also been used for fetal visualization to assist in the prenatal diagnosis of external malformations. However, ultrasound, with its improved resolution, has become a safer and more effective way to diagnose such abnormalities.

Direct fetal sampling is indicated when a family is at known high risk for producing an offspring with a handicapping or fatal disorder and there exists no other methodology for making a prenatal diagnosis (such as in the case of severe combined immunodeficiency disease). The public health impact of this technology is and probably shall remain small since it is being applied to diagnose a limited number of conditions in a few families.

Ultrasound Examination

Ultrasound imaging of body structure is based upon pulsed ultrasound (a nonionizing form of radiation) of high frequency and low intensity.[90,91] When the pulse encounters tissues of different density, the sound waves separate into components—part of which are reflected (seen as "echoes" by the transducer) and part of which continue onward. Scanning images can be portrayed simply as two-dimensional images.[90] As ultrasound technology has improved, its use as an adjunct to pregnancy management has soared. A California birth certificate survey found that a minimum of 15% of all pregnancies had one or more ultrasound examinations in 1978, while 75% of patients delivering a nonmalformed infant at Brigham & Women's Hospital in 1984 had one or more ultrasound scans.[92,93] A recent review of experimental animal and human ultrasound literature documented no short-term adverse effects ascribable to currently used diagnostic ultrasound in human fetuses.[92]

Ultrasound imaging has improved management of pregnancy with regard to: (1) determination of gestational age; (2) diagnosis of multiple gestations; (3) evaluation of fetal growth and well being; (4) evaluation of vaginal bleeding; and

(5) evaluation of size–date discrepancies (for additional indications see ref. 92).

Results from several randomized clinical trials of ultrasound use in pregnancy are becoming available. Although the study designs differ, it appears that pregnancies monitored by ultrasound studies have improved gestational dating and improved diagnosis of small-for-dates infants, large-for-dates infants, multiple gestations, and malformed infants.[92,94,95] Preliminary data from the largest study to date showed a trend toward decreased perinatal mortality and morbidity (that was not statistically significant) among the group receiving scans.[96]

The accuracy of ultrasound study for diagnosis of congenital malformations has not been evaluated systematically. There are multiple case reports and series demonstrating that ultrasound examination can diagnose successfully many fetal anomalies in virtually all body systems and organs.[90,97] It has even been suggested that all pregnancies be scanned to screen for fetal anomalies, especially neural tube defects.[98] However, the limitations of ultrasound accuracy have not been fully defined. Our data on the ultrasound diagnosis of intracranial anomalies shows that diagnostic accuracy is low for rare intracranial anomalies (such as holoprosencephaly and hydranencephaly) and is even lower for the presence of associated extracranial malformations.[99] Furthermore, accuracy depends on the experience of the operator and the quality of equipment being used. Finally, there have been no attempts to evaluate the cost–benefit ratio of routine ultrasound studies.

Maternal Blood Sampling

Prenatally diagnosing the presence of a malformed fetus on the basis of maternal blood or serum analysis is an optimistic, although not entirely unrealistic, goal. The potential for such methodology is great as it would offer no risk to the mother and the fetus, be applicable to many or all pregnancies, have the sample obtainable by untrained workers, and the entire diagnostic process might be very cost effective. Use of maternal serum alpha-fetoprotein (MSAFP) for the detection of NTDs is a prime example of this approach. Also, research is under way to selectively obtain fetal cells from the maternal circulation for prenatal diagnosis purposes.

Maternal serum alpha-fetoprotein (MSAFP)

High MSAFP Since the early reports demonstrating an association between elevated MSAFP and the presence of fetuses affected with NTDs,[100,101] the accuracy and reliability of this screening test has been evaluated rigorously. Detection of an elevated MSAFP leads to further diagnostic studies to rule in or out the presence of a malformation.

The manner in which AFP becomes elevated in the maternal serum in the presence of a fetus with an NTD is not precisely known. Normally during pregnancy, MSAFP levels are a 1000-fold lower than AFAFP levels.[27] AFP entry into the maternal circulation appears to be transplacental, but a small portion may transfer across the amniotic membranes as well.[61] Elevated amniotic fluid levels usually result in elevated maternal serum levels.

MSAFP begins to rise at approximately 13 weeks of gestation and peaks at about 32 weeks; this pattern is contrary to the amniotic fluid pattern which shows a steady decline after the end of the first trimester.[27] These discrepant patterns are not fully understood but may reflect rapid amniotic fluid volume expansion.[61]

A large prospective multicenter trial of MSAFP screening in the United Kingdom has demonstrated that an elevated MSAFP (specifically greater than 2.5 "multiples of the median" or MOM) has a sensitivity of 88% for the detection of fetuses with anencephaly and 79% for the detection of fetuses with open spina bifida.[102] The false-negative rates are 12 and 21%, respectively. Incomplete detection occurs because of the presence of overlap between the ranges of "normal" and "abnormal"; the overlap is considerable for both anencephaly and spina bifida but is more marked for spina bifida.[65]

Using the cutoff point of 2.5 MOM, 3.3% of non-NTD singleton pregnancies had elevated MSAFP (which constitutes a false-positive rate of 3.3%). Efforts to enhance the detection rate by lowering the cutoff point to 2.0 MOM doubles the false-positive rate.[102] It is important to point out that these detection frequencies are derived on a cohort of all pregnancies, not just pregnancies at high risk for a NTD. Many studies in other geographical regions (including three in the United States) report similar detection frequencies for open NTDs when screened at the optimal gestational age.[103–105] The false-positive rates on initial serum analysis are between 1 and 5% of all pregnancies screened; repeat analysis upon a fresh blood sample generally drops the false-positive rate by 20–50%.[65,103,105,106] There are many causes of elevated MSAFP besides NTDs (Table 7-5).

Elevations in MSAFP can be used as accurate screen for NTDs. However, it is a nonspecific marker. In fact, 90–95%

Table 7-5
Causes of MSAFP* > 2.5 × MOM*

Diagnosis	Frequency (%) of all pregnancies with MSAFP > 2.5 × MOM
Healthy singleton	40–60[61,105,106†]
Existing or impending fetal loss (SAB and NND)‡	9–17[61,105,106]
Multiple pregnancy	12–19[61,105,106]
Open NTDs	5–10[61,105,106]
Low birth weight	5.6–7.7[61,105]
Non-NTD congenital malformations (eg, abdominal-wall defects)	5[65,105,106]

*MSAFP, maternal serum alpha-fetoprotein; MOM, multiples of the median.
†At least 20% attributable to underestimate of gestational age.[27]
‡SAB = Spontaneous abortion; NND = Neonatal death.

of pregnancies found to have an elevated MSAFP level on initial screening will not have a fetus affected with a NTD[107] (but rather one of the outcomes listed in Table 7-5). Despite its low specificity, MSAFP screening programs are widespread in the United Kingdom. The UK average prevalence rate of 4.5 NTD cases/1000 births, the centralized health care system, and the economic benefits demonstrated by several studies all contribute to the program's implementation and continued existence.[61,102,108]

Large-scale MSAFP screening programs do not currently exist in North America despite study data demonstrating detection rates and false-positive rates comparable to those of the UK studies.[103,105] Lack of implementation appears to center on the generally lower prevalence of NTDs in the United States (1.5–1.75 cases/1000 births).[81,109] This lower prevalence affects the sensitivity in that an even smaller proportion of pregnancies with elevated MSAFP will actually have a fetus affected with a NTD[107] and also that a higher number of "unnecessary" amniocenteses will be performed.[110] Additional concerns are the lack of centralized medical care,[105] increasing the burden on already strained genetic counseling and laboratory facilities,[111] and the low diagnostic specificity of the screening test with its identification of many nonpreventable conditions. For example, in the case of an elevated MSAFP, the caretaker becomes aware that the pregnancy is at higher risk for having an adverse outcome such as a fetal loss or a low-birth-weight infant. However, the caretaker lacks the ability to identify which of these high-risk pregnancies will actually suffer from an adverse outcome.

Two studies have demonstrated that MSAFP screening can be cost effective even in areas of relatively low prevalence.[109,111] Both studies based calculations on a screening test with a high sensitivity, a high specificity, and 80–100% participation in the program, respectively. Despite feasibility, economic and humane justification (such cost–benefit analyses take no account of the avoided human suffering), widespread implementation of MSAFP programs in the United States may not occur unless additional benefits of screening can be documented.

Low MSAFP Since MSAFP values follow a normal distribution, approximately 50% of the values fall above the median and 50% below the median. Values that are considered "low" (<0.4 MOM or <0.25 MOM) are usually associated with a normal pregnancy outcome. The explanation for the low value can be attributed to an overestimate of gestational age in many cases.[112] However, low MSAFP has also been linked to subsequent fetal loss in several studies.[112–114] The most recent study showed that 59 of 155 pregnancies (38%) with MSAFP <0.25 MOM ended in a fetal loss.[112] The remaining 96 of 155 pregnancies (62%) had normal pregnancy outcomes. Both the etiology of the losses and the etiology of the low MSAFP level (in the presence of a live fetus at testing) remain unexplained.

An additional association between low MSAFP and aneuploidy has been suggested. Three studies have found a higher frequency of low MSAFP in pregnancies where the fetus is affected with trisomy 21 (Table 7-6). These three reports demonstrate that 80–84% of trisomy 21 pregnancies studied had MSAFP below the median; by definition, 50% of all pregnancies should fall below the median. Fifteen to 28%

Table 7-6
Cases of Trisomy 21 with Low MSAFP*

Study	No. Cases	Number of Cases			Normals <0.4 MOM
		<1.0 MOM	*<0.4 MOM*	*<0.25 MOM*	
Merkatz et al[78]	25	21 (84%)	7 (28%)	3 (12%)	(2.3–11.2%)
Cuckle et al[115]	61	49 (80%)	9 (15%)	2 (3.2%)	(4.4%)
Tabor et al[116]	25	21 (84%)			

*MSAFP, maternal serum alpha-fetoprotein; MOM, multiples of the median.

of cases had MSAFP <0.4 MOM in comparison to 4–11% of controls. The number of cases falling below 0.25 MOM is too small for informative comparisons. In these three reports, the average MSAFP level is lower in the trisomy 21 pregnancies than in control pregnancies, but this has not been confirmed in a fourth study.[78,115,116,117] Some reduction of AFAFP in trisomy 21 pregnancies has also been reported.[115,117,118]

There is little available data to evaluate the relationship of MSAFP to other chromosomal anomalies, but one study has found that 15 of 16 trisomy 13 and trisomy 18 pregnancies had MSAFP below the median, and that three of 16 (19%) had levels <0.4 MOM.[78]

It has been suggested that low MSAFP replace advanced maternal age as an indication for amniocentesis. As previously mentioned, by currently offering amniocentesis to women over 35 years of age, potentially 5% of the pregnant population receives an amniocentesis to identify 20–25% of trisomy 21 births.[78] Furthermore, the detection rate on this basis is 1–2 abnormalities/100 amniocenteses. Use of MSAFP screening may increase this detection frequency.[78]

MSAFP screening has appeal in being more "democratic"; that is, trisomy 21 could be detected in pregnancies across all maternal age groups. However, use of such a screening program for detection of chromosomal anomalies has certain problems. Since it would be used as a screening test, a cutoff point must be established to maximize the detection rate while minimizing the false-positive and false-negative rates. If one uses the median as the cutoff, 80–84% of trisomy 21 cases could theoretically be identified (after subsequent amniocentesis and karyotyping), but approximately 50% of all pregnancies would have to undergo amniocentesis. This same cutoff would falsely reassure 16–20% of women that their pregnancies would not be affected. Lowering the cutoff to 0.4 MOM would only lead to a maximal detection of 25% of cases and potentially 10% of all pregnancies would undergo amniocentesis to achieve this detection rate.

Low MSAFP, alone, appears too nonspecific to be considered a useful screening tool. Perhaps a sliding scale of MSAFP in conjunction with maternal age, as has been suggested by Cuckle et al,[115] will prove more sensitive and specific. Yet, no study has evaluated the frequency of all outcomes seemingly associated with low MSAFP. It is possible that the majority of pregnancies so identified will be normal or will have a nonpreventable outcome (such as spontaneous abortion) and that only a minority will potentially have an outcome for which intervention is appropriate or available. Therefore, it seems premature to offer this as a wide-scale screening program without further evaluation of (1) detection rates, false-positive rates, and false-negative rates for all detectable chromosomal abnormalities; (2) cost effectiveness, especially in combination with NTD screening; and (3) availability of cytogenetic facilities to handle additional analyses that will be required.

Fetal Blood Cells in Maternal Circulation

There is ongoing research to use fetal blood cells present in maternal circulation for prenatal diagnosis purposes. Maternal and fetal cells can be differentially radiolabeled and then separated by a fluorescent-activated cell sorter.[119] Currently, this technique can be used for Y-chromatin determination, but ultimately these cells might be cultured for chromosomal and biochemical analyses. At present, there is no public health impact.

PREVENTION OF MAJOR MALFORMATIONS

There are currently several situations in which the occurrence of malformations can be prevented. Since it is known that structural fetal development is essentially complete by the end of the embryonic period of gestation, prevention of a malformation must take place prior to conception or prior to the formation of a given organ or system during the first trimester.[120]

Prevention by Control or Elimination of a Causal Factor

Following the suggestion that nutritional deficiencies may contribute to the development of NTDs, several small British studies reported that either multivitamin supplementation and/or folic acid supplementation significantly reduced the recurrence rate of NTDs.[121,122] Small sample sizes and methodologic problems have prompted additional large-scale, well-designed trials to test this hypothesis.[123] Similar studies, one case–control in design and the other a recurrence trial, are being planned for the United States (where contributory etiologic factors may differ in a low-prevalence region) (J. Mills and L. Sever, personal communication).

Also included under this approach is avoidance of known or suspected teratogenic agents or substances such as ionizing radiation, teratogenic drugs, and certain environmental or chemical substances.[2,124] Although certain agents may be successfully avoided during the first trimester, such as the possibility of temporarily discontinuing phenytoin use in an epileptic patient, most of such exposures occur unknowingly. This general approach of factor elimination or control has appeal on many grounds, prime among which is its potential ease of applicability. However, current ignorance about significant causal factors limits the impact of this approach.

Prevention by Eradication of Maternal Disease

The prime example of this approach is the prevention of rubella infection by vaccination. Maternal infection with rubella virus during the first trimester of pregnancy produces a high rate of fetal anomalies, especially of the ocular, auditory, cardiac, and central nervous systems.[125] The characteristic pattern of malformations has been called the congenital rubella syndrome (CRS). Between 1969, the time of introduction of the rubella vaccine into the United States, and 1981, the reported cases of rubella have declined by 96% and only 10 cases of CRS were reported to the Centers for Disease Control in 1981.[126] CRS has not been eliminated from either the United States or the United Kingdom, with approximately 10–20% of women in the reproductive years susceptible to rubella. Intensified efforts to vaccinate both young children and teenaged women may successfully eradicate any malformation burden attributable to rubella. There exist no other maternal diseases or infections which can be currently eliminated or eradicated by wide-scale vaccination programs.

Prevention by Control of Maternal Disease

A number of adverse reproductive outcomes, including major malformations, can be reduced by improved management of certain maternal diseases or conditions. Prime examples are listed below.

Maternal phenylketonuria Maternal hyperphenylalaninemia has been shown to have adverse effects on the developing fetus. Reported adverse effects include low birth weight, congenital heart disease, microcephaly, and mental retardation.[127] Higher maternal serum levels have been most strongly linked with reduced intellectual performance in the offspring.[128] Preconceptual dietary manipulation in an attempt to bring maternal phenylalanine levels to the range of normal may lessen the risk of fetal adverse effects.[129]

Maternal diabetes mellitus The rate of major malformations among offspring of diabetics is two- to threefold higher than among offspring of nondiabetics.[130] Poor diabetic control, as manifested by elevated hemoglobin Alc in early pregnancy, is associated with an increased risk of major malformations.[131] Aggressive dietary and insulin management prior to conception and during early pregnancy to maintain normoglycemia has been reported to lead to a significant reduction in the risk of major malformations.[132,133]

Maternal alcoholism The triad of prenatal and/or postnatal growth retardation, characteristic craniofacial dysmorphology, and central nervous system dysfunction has been labeled the fetal alcohol syndrome (FAS).[134,135] There may be an increase in the frequency of major malformations as well.[134] Although these are a nonspecific constellation of findings, they have been reported in the offspring of chronic alcoholic women of differing ethnic and social class backgrounds. A dose–response effect has not been consistently demonstrated in studies of human populations, but FAS is usually reported in the presence of moderate or heavy alcohol intake throughout pregnancy.[136] However, it is important to note that the physical features of FAS have been observed in the offspring of moderate drinkers in early pregnancy, and there even exists a case report of FAS in an offspring of former alcoholic parents.[137,138] It does appear that cessation or moderation of drinking in the second or third trimester reduces the amount of alcohol-induced growth retardation.[139]

Prevention Prior to Conception

A couple at known high risk for producing a malformed offspring (generally on the basis of a positive family history or a previously affected offspring) may elect adoption, rather than conception, or conception via artificial insemination.[124]

CONCLUSIONS

Prenatal detection of malformed fetuses is the primary method available at the present time to reduce the prevalence of malformed newborns. To expand the public health impact of these methods, further investigations are required.

Specifically, the accuracy and cost effectiveness of routine ultrasound examination for the diagnosis of congenital malformations needs to be established prior to any recommendation of routine ultrasound screening. Likewise, evaluation of the sensitivity, specificity, and cost effectiveness of screening programs identifying pregnancies with either low or high MSAFP levels is necessary prior to the development of any large-scale programs in the United States.

Unfortunately, prenatal detection takes place most often in the second trimester and consequently, couples are often faced with difficult decisions about pregnancy termination. Preventing the development of malformations has far greater humane, medical, and economic appeal. Questions about the effectiveness of periconceptual vitamin supplementation in reducing the occurrence and recurrence of NTDs need to be resolved. Research of other possible prevention strategies needs strong support.

ACKNOWLEDGMENTS

I wish to thank Martha Werler and Sharon Kidd for helpful discussions in the preparation of this manuscript.

REFERENCES

1. Wegman ME: Annual summary of vital statistics—1983. *Pediatrics* 1984;74:981–990.
2. Kalter H, Warkany J: Congenital malformations: Etiologic factors and their role in prevention. *N Engl J Med* 1983;308:424–431,491–497.
3. Holmes LB, Vincent SE, Cook C, et al: *Surveillance of Newborn Infants For Malformations Due to Spontaneous Mutations. Population and Biological Aspects of Human Mutation.* New York, Academic Press, 1981.
4. Myrianthopoulos NC, Chung CS: Congenital malformations in singletons: Epidemiologic survey. *Birth Defects Original Article Series* 1974;X(11):1–58.
5. Marden PM, Smith DW, McDonald MJ: Congenital anomalies in the newborn infant including minor variations. *J Pediatr* 1964;64:357–371.

6. Fraser FC: Relation of animal studies to the problem in man, in Wilson JG, Fraser FC (eds): *Handbook of Teratology.* New York, Plenum Press, 1977, pp 75–96.
7. Lin CC, Gedeon MM, Griffith P, et al: Chromosome analysis on 930 consecutive newborn children using quinacrine fluorescent banding technique. *Hum Genet* 1976;31:315–328.
8. Buckton KE, O'Riordan ML, Ratcliffe S, et al: A G-band study of chromosomes in liveborn infants. *Ann Hum Genet* 1980;43:227–239.
9. Stene J, Stene E, Stengel-Rutkowski S, et al: Paternal age and Down's syndrome. *Hum Genet* 1981;59:119–124.
10. Neel JV: A study of major congenital defects in Japanese infants. *Am J Hum Genet* 1958;10:398–445.
11. Say B, Tunçbilek E, Balci S, et al: Incidence of congenital malformations in a sample of the Turkish population. *Hum Hered* 1973;23:434–441.
12. Simpkiss M, Lowe A: Congenital abnormalities in the African newborn. *Arch Dis Child* 1961;36:404–406.
13. Stewart AL, Keay AJ, Smith PG: Congenital malformations: A detailed study of 2500 liveborn infants. *Ann Hum Genet* 1969;32:353–360.
14. Emmanuel I, Huang SW, Gutman LT, et al: The incidence of congenital malformations in a Chinese population: The Taipei collaborative study. *Teratology* 1972;5:159–170.
15. Erickson JD: Racial variations in the incidence of congenital malformations. *Ann Hum Genet* 1976;39:315–320.
16. Harris LE, Stayura LA, Ramirez-Talavera PF, et al: Congenital and acquired abnormalities observed in live-born and stillborn neonates. *Mayo Clin Proc* 1975;50:85–90.
17. Niswander JD, Barrow MV, Bingle GJ: Congenital malformations in the American Indian. *Social Biol* 1975;22:203–215.
18. Drew JH, Parkinson P, Walstab JE, et al: Incidence and types of malformations in newborn infants. *Med J Aust* 1977;1: 945–949.
19. Leck I, Record RG, McKeown T, et al: The incidence of malformations in Birmingham, England, 1950–1959. *Teratology* 1968;1:263–280.
20. Elwood JM, Elwood JH: *Epidemiology of Anencephalus and Spina Bifida.* Oxford, England, Oxford University Press, 1980.
21. Sever LE: *Epidemiologic Aspects of Neural Tube Defects in Prevention of Neural Tube Defects.* New York, Academic Press, 1978.
22. Naggan L, MacMahon B: Ethnic differences in the prevalence

of anencephaly and spina bifida in Boston, Massachusetts. *N Engl J Med* 1967;277:1119–1123.
23. MacMahon B, Yen S: Unrecognized epidemic of anencephaly and spina bifida. *Lancet* 1971;1:31–34.
24. Aylett MJ, Roberts CJ, Lloyd S: Neural tube defects in a country town. *Br J Prev Soc Med* 1974;28:177–179.
25. Stein SC, Feldman JG, Friedlander M, et al: Is meningomyelocoele a disappearing disease? *Pediatrics* 1982;69:511–514.
26. Windham GC, Edmonds LD: Current trends in the incidence of neural tube defects. *Pediatrics* 1982;70:333–337.
27. Ferguson-Smith MA: The reduction of neural tube defects by maternal serum alpha-fetoprotein screening. *Br Med Bull* 1983;39:365–372.
28. Smithells RW, Sheppard S, Schorah CJ: Vitamin deficiencies and neural tube defects. *Arch Dis Child* 1976;51:944–949.
29. Fedrick J: Anencephalus in the Oxford record linkage study area. *Dev Med Child Neurol* 1976;18:643–656.
30. Hibbard ED, Smithells RW: Folic acid metabolism and human embryopathy. *Lancet* 1965;1:1254.
31. Rodeck CH, Morsman JM, Nicolaides KH, et al: A single operator technique for first trimester chorion biopsy. *Lancet* 1983;2:798.
32. Simoni G, Brambati B, Danesino C, et al: Efficient direct chromosome analysis and enzyme determination from chorionic villi samples in the first trimester of pregnancy. *Hum Genet* 1983;63:349.
33. Gosden JR, Mitchell AR, Gosden CM, et al: Direct vision chorion biopsy and chromosome-specified DNA probes for determination of fetal sex in the first trimester. *Lancet* 1982;2:1416.
34. Kazy Z, Rozovsky IS, Bakharev VA: Chorion biopsy in early pregnancy: A method of early prenatal diagnosis for inherited disorder. *Prenatal Diagnosis* 1981;2:39.
35. Old JM, Ward RHT, Petroum M, et al: First trimester diagnosis for haemoglobinopathies: Three cases. *Lancet* 1982;2:1413.
36. Kleijer WT, van Diggelen OP, Janse HC, et al: First trimester diagnosis of Hunter syndrome on chorionic villi. *Lancet* 1984;472.
37. Miller WA: Chorionic villus biopsy. *Genetic Resource (Commonwealth Mass)* 1984;1:2.
38. Simpson JL: Low fetal loss rate after normal ultrasound at eight weeks gestation: Implications for chorionic villus sampling (CVS). (Abstract) *Am J Hum Genet* 1984;36(S):197S.

39. Turnbull AC, MacKenzie IZ: Second trimester amniocentesis and termination of pregnancy. *Br Med Bull* 1983;39:315–321.
40. The NICHD national registry for amniocentesis group. Mid-trimester amniocentesis for prenatal diagnosis. *JAMA* 1976; 236:1471–1476.
41. Report to the Medical Research council by their working party on amniocentesis and assessment of the hazards of amniocentesis. *Br J Obstet Gynecol* 1978;85:(suppl).
42. Simpson NE, Dallaire L, Miller JR, et al: Prenatal diagnosis of genetic disease in Canada: Report of a collaborative study. *Can Med Assoc J* 1976;115:739–746.
43. Wald NJ, Terziani E, Vickers PA, et al: Congenital talipes and malformation in relation to amniocentesis: A case—control study. *Lancet* 1983;2:246–249.
44. Karp LE, Hayden PW: Fetal puncture during midtrimester amniocentesis. *Obstet Gynecol* 1977;49:115–117.
45. Rehder H, Weitzel H: Intrauterine amputations after amniocentesis. *Lancet* 1978;1:382.
45a. Stock RJ: Fetal death secondary to needle laceration during second trimester amniocentesis: A case report. *Prenatal Diagnosis* 1982;2:133–137.
46. Sandstrom MM, Beauchesne MT, Gustashaw KM, et al: Prenatal cytogenetic diagnosis. *Methods Cell Biol* 1982; 26:35–66.
47. Gosden CM: Amniotic fluid cell types and culture. *Br Med Bull* 1983;39:348–354.
48. Golbus MS, Loughman WD, Epstein CJ, et al: Prenatal genetic diagnosis in 3000 amniocenteses. *N Engl J Med* 1979; 300:157–163.
49. Ferguson-Smith MA: Prenatal chromosome analysis and its impact on the birth incidence of chromosome disorders. *Br Med Bull* 1983;39:355–364.
50. Grabowski GA, Desnick RJ: Prenatal diagnosis of inherited metabolic diseases: Principles, pitfalls, and prospects. *Methods Cell Biol* 1982;26:96–180.
51. Patrick AD: Inherited metabolic disorders. *Br Med Bull* 1983;39:378–385.
52. Orkin SH, Little PFR, Kazazian HH, et al: Improved detection of the sickle mutation by DNA analysis. *N Engl J Med* 1982;307:32–36.
53. Humphries SE, Williamson R: Application of recombinant DNA technology to prenatal detection of inherited defects. *Br Med Bull* 1983;39:343–347.

54. Boehm CD, Antonarakis SE, Phillips JA, et al: Prenatal diagnosis using DNA polymorphisms. *N Engl J Med* 1983; 308:1054–1058.
55. Woo SLC: Prenatal diagnosis and carrier detection of classic phenylketonuria by gene analysis. *Pediatrics* 1984;74:412–423.
56. Gusella JF, Wexler NS, Conneally PM, et al: A polymorphic DNA marker genetically linked to Huntington's Disease. *Nature* 1983;306:234–238.
57. Levine LS, Zachmann M, New MI, et al: Genetic mapping of the 21-hydroxylase deficiency gene within the HLA linkage group. *N Engl J Med* 1978;299:911–915.
58. Dupont B, Oberfield SE, Smithwick EM, et al: Close genetic linkage between HLA and congenital adrenal hyperplasia (21-hydroxylase deficiency) *Lancet* 1977;2:1309–1311.
59. Gitlin D, Boesman M: Sites of serum alpha fetoprotein synthesis in the human and in the rat. *J Clin Invest* 1967;46:1010–1016.
60. Haddow JE, Miller WA: Prenatal diagnosis of open neural tube defects. *Methods Cell Biol* 1982;26:68–95.
61. Wald NJ, Cuckle HS: Open neural tube defects in antenatal and neonatal screening, in Wald NJ (ed): *Neonatal and Antenatal Screening.* Oxford, England, Oxford University Press, 1984, pp 25–73.
62. Brock DJH: Amniotic fluid tests for fetal neural tube defects. *Br Med Bull* 1983;39:373–377.
63. Second report of the UK collaborative study on alpha-fetoprotein in relation to neural tube defects. Amniotic fluid alpha-fetoprotein measurement in antenatal diagnosis of anencephaly and open spina bifida in early pregnancy. *Lancet* 1979;2:651–662.
64. Wald NJ, Cuckle HS, Latz C, et al: Alpha-fetoprotein screening and diagnosis of fetal open neural tube defects: The need for quality control. *Am J Obstet Gynecol* 1981;141:1–4.
65. Fourth report of the UK collaborative study on alpha-fetoprotein in relation to neural tube defects. Estimating an individual's risk of having a fetus with open spina bifida and the value of repeat alpha-fetoprotein testing. *J Epidemiol Community Health* 1982;36:87–95.
66. Sceppala M, Ruoslahti E: Alpha-fetoprotein in antenatal diagnosis. *Lancet* 1973;1:155.
67. Milunsky A: Prenatal detection of neural tube defects: False positive and negative results. *Pediatrics* 1977;59:782–783.
68. Smith AD, Wald NJ, Cuckle HS, et al: Amniotic fluid

acetylcholinesterase as a possible diagnostic test for neural tube defects in early pregnancy. *Lancet* 1979;1:685–688.

69. Laurence KM: Clinical and ethical considerations on alphafetoprotein estimation for early prenatal diagnosis of neural tube malformations. *Dev Med Child Neurol (Suppl)* 1974; 32:117–121.
70. Brock DJH: Antenatal misdiagnosis of nerual tube defects. *Lancet* 1975;2:495.
71. Zeisel SH, Milunsky A, Blusztajn JK: Prenatal diagnosis of neural tube defects V. The value of amniotic fluid cholinesterase studies. *Am J Obstet Gynecol* 1980;137:481–485.
72. Report of the collaborative acetylcholinesterase study. Amniotic fluid acetylcholinesterase electrophoresis as a secondary test in the diagnosis of anencephaly and open spina bifida in early pregnancy. *Lancet* 1981;2:321–324.
73. Brock DJH: Prenatal diagnosis of cystic fibrosis using monoclonal antibodies specific for the isoenzyme of alkaline phosphatase. (Abstract) *Am J Hum Genet* 1984;36:1865.
74. Brock DJH, Hayward C: Prenatal diagnosis of cystic fibrosis by methylum belliferylguanidino benzoate protease titration in amniotic fluid. *Prenatal Diagnosis* 1983;3:1–5.

74a. Dann LG, Baker S, Grinham C, et al: Calcium concentration in the prenatal diagnosis of cystic fibrosis. *Prenatal Diagnosis* 1983;3:161–164.

75. Turnbull AC, MacKenzie IZ: Second-trimester amniocentesis and termination of pregnancy. *Br Med Bull* 1983;39:315–321.
76. New England Regional Genetics Group; Amniocentesis Survey—1984.
77. Galjaard H: European experience with prenatal diagnosis of congenital disease: A survey of 6121 cases. *Cytogenet Cell Genet* 1976;16:453–467.
78. Merkatz IR, Nitowsky HM, Macri JN, et al: An association between low maternal serum alpha-fetoprotein and fetal chromosomal abnormalities. *Am J Obstet Gynecol* 1984;148: 886–892.
79. Stene J, Mikkelson M: Down syndrome and other chromosome disorders in antenatal and neonatal screening, in Wald NJ (ed): *Neonatal and Antenatal Screening.* Oxford, England, Oxford University Press, 1984, pp 74–105.
80. Hook EB, Schreinemachers DM: Trends in utilization of prenatal cytogenetic diagnosis by New York State residents in 1979 and 1980. *Am J Public Health* 1983;73:198–202.
81. Sadovnick AD, Baird PA: A cost benefit analysis of prenatal

detection of Down syndrome and neural tube defects in older mothers. *Am J Med Genet* 1981;10:367–378.

82. Hagard S, Carter FA: Preventing the birth of infants with Down's syndrome: Cost–benefit analysis. *Br Med J* 1976;1: 753–756.
83. Jackson-Cook CK, Flannery DB, Corey LA, et al: The double NOR variant: A risk factor in trisomy 21. (Abstract) *Am J Hum Genet* 1984;36:97S.
84. Rodeck CH: Fetoscopy and fetal blood sampling in antenatal and neonatal screening, in Wald NJ (ed): *Neonatal and Antenatal Screening.* Oxford, England, Oxford University Press, 1984;457–479.
85. Rodeck CH, Kemp JR, Holman LA, et al: Direct intravascular fetal blood transfusion by fetoscopy in severe rhesus isoimmunization. *Lancet* 1981;1:625–627.
86. Rodeck LH, Nicolaides KH: Fetoscopy and fetal tissue sampling. *Br Med Bull* 1983;39:332–337.
87. Elias S, Esterly NB: Prenatal diagnosis of hereditary skin disorders. *Clin Obstet Gynecol* 1981;24:1069–1087.
88. Rodeck LH, Patrick AD, Pembrey ME, et al: Fetal liver biopsy for prenatal diagnosis of ornithine carbamyl transferase deficiency. *Lancet* 1982;2:297–299.
89. Nicolaides KH, Koullapis EN, Rodeck CH: The safety of fetoscopy: (II) Effect on maternal plasma levels of 13,14-dihydro-15-oxoprostaglandin $F_{2\alpha}$. *Prenatal Diagnosis* 1983;3:97–100.
90. Campbell S, Griffin D, Little D, et al: Use of ultrasound in the prenatal diagnosis of congenital disorders. *Methods Cell Biol* 1982;26:181–228.
91. Pizzarello DJ: Teratogenic effects of ionizing radiation and ultrasound. *Prog Clin Biol Res* 1979;44:67–76.
92. US Department of Health and Human Services, Public Health Services, National Institutes of Health. *Diagnostic Ultrasound Imaging in Pregnancy.* NIH Publication No 84:667,1984.
93. Homes LB: *Malformation Surveillance.* Brigham & Women's Hospital, 1984, unpublished data.
94. Wladimiroff JW, Laar J: Ultrasonic measurement of fetal body size: A randomized controlled trial. *Acta Obstet Gynecol Scand* 1980;59:177–179.
95. Eik-Nes SH, Økland O: *Ultrasound Screening of Pregnant Women—a Prospective Randomized Study.* NIH Publication No 84:667,1984.
96. Eik-Nes SH, Økland O, Aure JC, et al: Ultrasound screening

in pregnancy: A randomized controlled trial. *Lancet* 1984; 1:1347.

97. Campbell S, Pearce JM: Ultrasound visualization of congenital malformations. *Br Med Bull* 1983;39:322–331.
98. Harris R, Read AP: New uncertainties in prenatal screening for neural tube defect. *Br Med J* 1981;282:1416–1418.
99. Pober BR, Green MF, Holmes LB: Complexities of hydrocephalus. *Teratology* 1984;29:51A.
100. Sellen MJ, Singer JD, Coltart TM, et al: Maternal serum alphafetoprotein levels and prenatal diagnosis of neural-tube defects. *Lancet* 1974;1:428–429.
101. Brock DJH, Bolton AE, Monaghan JM: Prenatal diagnosis of anencephaly through maternal serum alpha fetoprotein measurement. *Lancet* 1973;2:923–924.
102. Report of UK Collaborative Study on alpha-fetoprotein in relation to neural tube defects. Maternal serum alpha-fetoprotein measurement in antenatal screening for anencephaly and spina bifida in early pregnancy. *Lancet* 1977;1:1323–1332.
103. Gardner S, Burton BK, Johnson AM: Maternal serum alphafetoprotein screening: A report of the Forsyth County Project. *Am J Obstet Gynecol* 1981;140:250–253.
104. Macri JN: Current status of alpha-fetoprotein prenatal testing. *Prog Clin Biol Res* 1979;44:47–63.
105. Milunsky A, Alpert E: Results and benefits of maternal serum alpha-fetoprotein screening program. *JAMA* 1984;252: 1438–1442.
106. Kjessler B, Johansson SGO: Monitoring of the development of early pregnancy by determination of alpha-fetoprotein in maternal serum and amniotic fluid samples. *Acta Obstet Gynecol Scand (Suppl)* 1977;69:5–14.
107. Wald NJ: Workgroup paper. The interpretation of AFP values and the effect of AFP assay performance on screening efficacy in maternal serum alpha-fetoprotein. Proceedings of a conference held by the National Center for Health Care Technology and the Food and Drug Administration. Gaskel B, Haddow JE, Fletcher JC, Neal A: (eds) 1980:29–33.
108. Hagard S, Carter F, Milne RG: Screening for spina bifida cystica. *Br J Prev Soc Med* 1976;30:40–53.
109. Layde PM, von Allman SD, Oakley GP: Maternal serum alphafetoprotein screening: A cost-benefit analysis. *Am J Public Health* 1979;69:566–573.
110. Brock DJH: Prenatal diagnosis—chemical methods. *Br Med Bull* 1978;32:16–20.

111. Sadovnick AD, Baird PA: A cost–benefit analysis of a population screening programme for neural tube defects. *Prenatal Diagnosis* 1983;3:117–126.
112. Davenport DM, Macri JN: The clinical significance of low maternal serum alpha-fetoprotein. *Am J Obstet Gynecol* 1983;146:657–661.
113. Kjessler B, Johansson SGO, Lidbjork G, et al: Alphafetoprotein (AFP) levels in maternal serum in relation to pregnancy outcome in 7158 pregnant women prospectively investigated during their 14th–20th week post last menstrual period. *Acta Obstet Gynecol Scand (Suppl)* 1977;69:25–44.
114. Lidbjork G, Kjessler B, Johansson SGO: Alpha-fetoprotein (AFP) levels in maternal serum in 115 patients with spontaneous abortion. *Acta Obstet Gynecol Scand (Suppl)* 1977;69:50–53.
115. Cuckle HS, Wald NJ, Lindenbaum RH: Maternal serum alphafetoprotein measurement: A screening test for Down's syndrome. *Lancet* 1984;1:926–929.
116. Tabor A, Norgaard-Pederson B, Jacobsen JC: Low maternal serum AFP and Down syndrome. *Lancet* 1984;2:161.
117. Cowchock FS, Ruch DA: Letter. *Lancet* 1984;2:161–162.
118. Trigg ME, Hitchens J, Geier MR, et al: Letter. *Lancet* 1984;2:161.
119. Parks DR, Herzenberg LA: Fetal cells from maternal blood: Their selection and prospects for use in prenatal diagnosis. *Methods Cell Biol* 1982;26:278–295.
120. Patten BM: *Human Embryology.* New York, McGraw-Hill Book Company, 1968.
121. Laurence KM, Nansi J, Miller MH, et al: Double-blind randomized control trial of folate supplement before conception to prevent recurrence of neural tube defects. *Br Med J* 1981;282:1509–1511.
122. Smithells RW, Sheppard S, Schorah CJ, et al: Possible prevention of neural-tube defects by periconceptual vitamin supplementation. *Lancet* 1980;1:339–340.
123. Beardsley T: MRC folate trials to start at last. *Nature* 1983;303:647.
124. Galjaard H: Early diagnosis and prevention of genetic disease: Molecules and the obstetrician, in Scrimgeour JB (ed): *Towards the Prevention of Fetal Malformation.* Edinburgh University Press, 1978, pp 3–19.
125. McIntosh K: Viral infections of the fetus and newborn, in Avery ME, Taeusch HW (eds): *Diseases of the Newborn.* Philadelphia, W.B. Saunders Co, 1984; pp 754–768.

126. Recommendations of the Immunization Practices Advisory Committee. Rubella Prevention. Morbidity and Mortality Weekly Report 1984;33(22):301–317.
127. Lenke RR, Levy HL: Maternal phenylketonuria and hyperphenylalaninemia: An international survey of the outcome of untreated and treated pregnancies. *N Engl J Med* 1980; 303:1202–1208.
128. Levy HL, Waisbren SE: Effects of untreated maternal phenylketonuria and hyperphenylalaninemia. *N Engl J Med* 1983;309:1269–1274.
129. Lenke RR, Levy HL: Maternal phenylketonuria—results of dietary therapy. *Am J Obstet Gynecol* 1982;142:548–553.
130. Gabbe SG, Mestman JH, Freeman RK: Management and outcome of pregnancy in diabetes mellitus, classes B to R. *Am J Obstet Gynecol* 1977;129:723–729.
131. Miller E, Hare JW, Cloherty JP, et al: Elevated maternal hemoglobin Alc in early pregnancy and major congenital anomalies in infants of diabetic mothers. *N Engl J Med* 1981;304:1331–1334.
132. Fuhrman K, Reiher H, Semmler K, et al: Prevention of congenital malformations in the infants of insulin dependent diabetic mothers. *Diabetes Care* 1983;6:219–223.
133. Tevaarwerk GJM, Harding PGR, Milne KJ, et al: Pregnancy in diabetic women: Outcome with a program aimed at normoglycemia before meals. *Can Med Assoc J* 1981;125:435–442.
134. Clarren SK, Smith DW: The fetal alcohol syndrome. *N Engl J Med* 1978;298:1063–1067.
135. Jones KL, Smith DW, Ulleland CN, et al: Pattern of malformation in offspring of chronic alcoholic mothers. *Lancet* 1973;1:1267–1271.
136. Little RE, Graham JM, Samson HH: Fetal alcohol effects in humans and animals. *Adv Alcohol Substance Abuse* 1982;1:103–125.
137. Hanson JW, Streissguth AP, Smith DW: The effects of moderate alcohol consumption during pregnancy on fetal growth and morphogenesis. *J Pediatr* 1978;92:457–460.
138. Scheiner AP, Donovan CM, Bartoshesky LE: Fetal alcohol syndrome in a child whose parents had stopped drinking. *Lancet* 1979;1:1077–1078.
139. Rosett HL, Weiner L, Zuckerman B, et al: Reduction of alcohol consumption during pregnancy with benefits to the newborn. *Alcoholism* 1980;4:178–183.

Eastern College of Nursing Library

Appendix
Prevalence Rate of Selected Malformations (Rate/1000 Births)

Apparent etiology	Specific example	US Whites[4*] (*N* = 24,153)	US Blacks[4*] (*N* = 25,126)	Japan[10] (*N* = 64,569)
Genetic abnormalities				
Chromosomal	Trisomy 21	2.4	1.9	0.09
Monogenic				
"Familial"	Postaxial polydactyly	3.5	27.8	0.60
Multifactorial inheritance				
	Anencephaly and spina bifida	2.0	0.48	0.82
	Cleft lip and palate	5.4	3.3	2.7
	Congenital heart disease	–[†]	–	1.5
Environmental factors				
Maternal condition	Diabetes mellitus	–	–	–
Intrauterine infection	CMV	0	–	–
Teratogenic drugs	Phenytoin	–	–	–
Unknown Cause				
	Intestinal atresia	0.03	0	0.03
	Diaphragmatic hernia	0.25	0.16	0.03
Method of Ascertainment		Prospective examination of infants:		
		Infant	Infant	Infant
Years of study		1959–1966	1959–1966	1948–1954

*US Collaborative Perinatal Project. Higher prevalence rates due to ascertainment up to 1 year of age.
†Outcome not studied or insufficient information.
‡MACDP = Metropolitan Atlanta Congenital Defects Program.

Turkey[11] (N = 9947)	Uganda[12] (N = 2068)	Scotland[13] (N = 2500)	Taipei[14] (N = 25,814)	Georgia[15] Whites (N = 121,900)
0.70	0.50	1.2	0.6	–
2.3	13.5	1.2	1.8	1.2
3.0	0	1.2	1.4	2.4
1.1	1.4	1.2	3.9	1.7
1.7	0.5	2.0	–	–
–	–	–	–	–
–	–	–	–	–
–	–	–	–	–
–	0.5	0	0.7	–
–	–	1.2	–	–
Prospective examination of infants:			Prospective exam of selected infants	Prospective surveillance of nurseries MACDP‡
Infant 1969	Infant 1956–1957	Infant 1965–1967	1965–1968	1967–1973

Appendix (continued)

Georgia[15] Blacks (N = 48,700)	Minnesota[16] (N = 21,442)	US Indian[17] (N = 43,711)	Australia[18] (N = 10,454)	England[19] (N = 190,236)
–	1.5	0.9	1.2	1.1
11.0	0.9	2.1	0.67	1.0
0.90	1.5	0.9	2.8	4.77
1.0	1.5	2.4	2.6	1.7
–	3.0	2.8	5.8	2.2
–	–	–	–	–
–	–	–	–	–
–	–	–	–	–
–	0.7	0.34	0.4	0.26
–	0.09	0.20	0.6	0.13
Prospective surveillance of nurseries MACDP‡	Review of hospital records and vital statistics			
1967–1973	1951–1963	1964–1969	1971–1975	1950–1959

CHAPTER 8

REPRODUCTION AND THE WORKING ENVIRONMENT

Michael Rosenberg, MD, MPH

INTRODUCTION

Today's United States work force includes some 109 million men and women between the ages of 15 and 44 who work with an estimated 70,000 chemical, biological, and physical agents.[1] Only a small fraction of these agents have been evaluated in humans for their reproductive toxicity, but several dramatic episodes of reproductive problems attributable to exposure leave little doubt that chemical, physical, and biological agents used in the workplace can exert powerful adverse effects on the ability to reproduce. Recent evidence also suggests that many reproductive problems traditionally associated with women, such as spontaneous fetal loss, have a component attributable to toxic exposures to men.

The magnitude of reproductive problems attributable to occupation cannot be gauged with presently available data. The relationship between occupation and reproduction has nonetheless become a prominent concern over the past decade for three reasons.[1] First, the number of women in the work force has been increasing in both absolute and relative terms: in 1970, women comprised 38% of the work force; by 1978, the proportion rose to 42%; and by 1990, women are expected to compose 46% of the work force. Second, demographic trends of decreasing numbers of children in each family and women's later age at first birth are focusing increasing attention on assuring that children are born healthy. Third, health care systems of industrialized nations have evolved from concern with diseases of poverty, malnutrition, and poor personal hygiene to scrutiny of health impairments due to the environment and occupation.

This chapter has two goals: first, to review recognized and suspected occupational influences on reproduction and their clinical implications, and second, to discuss methodological issues that affect the way studies are conducted and interpreted. Because the study of occupation and reproduction is relatively new, studies that clearly indicate how an occupational exposure affects reproduction are few. This new discipline also lacks established methodology and definition of terms; thus, emphasis will be placed on these points as they pertain to past and future research. This chapter will emphasize chemical exposures which occur in the workplace; the reader may wish to consult other references for effects of physical or biological agents.

OCCUPATIONAL HISTORY

Although it is often said that the importance of a good clinical history cannot be overstated, this adage is probably nowhere as true as it is for the clinician evaluating the effect of occupation. The clinician faces several problems: first, exposures to toxic agents may affect reproduction without clinical signs that might provide clues to unusual exposures. Second, patients are often poorly informed about the specific chemical, physical, and biological agents they work with. Third, many common agents are incompletely studied, or not studied at all, in humans. Clinicians may see patients with common exposures and reproductive problems infrequently enough that an association between the two may not occur to them. The clinician's difficulty is increased when one considers the inadequate training in occupational problems generally provided and the dearth of material on occupational impairments available to physicians. For these reasons, every clinical history should include these factors:[2]

1. Description of all jobs held. This should include job title and the duties actually performed.
2. Suspected and known hazardous work exposures. Each chemical has a product safety summary available from the manufacturer, and this may be consulted. Workers often know many of the agents with which they work.
3. Protective measures used.
4. Patterns of symptoms or illnesses among fellow workers.
5. Non-work-related environmental and other exposures. Smoking, alcohol, and age are the most important factors affecting reproductive ability for both men and women.

Most occupational agents that are recognized as impairing reproduction were first identified through observations by astute clinicians. Thus, the need for a careful clinical approach is also important both for present workers and for future patients and physicians who may profit from careful clinical attention. This is particularly important because the high number of agents being used and large numbers of persons using them are likely to result in the identification of additional associations.

Observations of unusual events (case reports) are generally followed by analytic studies. An analytic study is one that includes a group of nonexposed persons (control subjects) and compares the frequency of an outcome measure (some aspect of impaired reproduction, such as rate of spontaneous abortion) in this group with a similar group of persons exposed to a suspected agent. How studies are performed and how they are evaluated are important to clinicians because of the need to judge their merits and weaknesses in determining advice and treatment for patients. For that reason, and also because the great number of agents used and persons exposed raises the possibility that a physician may identify additional associations, a brief guide to assessing occupational studies follows.

ASSESSING REPRODUCTIVE IMPAIRMENTS

Although a long list of reproductive impairments have been described, they fall into three groups: impaired fecundability, or difficulty in becoming pregnant; increased rates of pregnancy loss; and birth or developmental disorders (Table 8-1).

Infecundability

Indices used to gauge the ability to become pregnant include infertility and time to conceive. Both imply a desire to become pregnant. The National Center for Health Statistics indicates that the overall rate of impaired fecundability among American couples (those married couples of reproductive age desiring a pregnancy but unable to achieve one) is approximately 16%.[3] The term infertility is used clinically to denote the lack of conception after one year of unprotected intercourse. (Demographers refer to inability to conceive as infecundability.)

This measure is generally applied retrospectively and is somewhat crude in that it fails to consider frequency and intermittent or partial use of contraceptives. The second measure is time to conceive, which is the interval between cessation of contraception and conception. This measure is generally used in prospective studies and can be a highly specific and reliable index. Its limitation is that this kind of information is difficult to ascertain retrospectively with

Table 8-1
End Points for Study of Reproductive Function*

Infecundability
1. Sexual dysfunction: libido, potency
2. Sperm abnormalities: number, motility, morphology
3. Amenorrhea
4. Anovulatory menstrual cycles
5. Infertility
6. Time to conceive

Fetal loss
1. Early (≤2500 g)
2. Late (28+ weeks)

Birth or developmental disorders
1. Intrapartum death
2. Low birth weight (<2500 g)
3. Birth defects: major, minor
4. Chromosomal abnormalities
5. Death in first week of life
6. Death in first month of life
7. Death in first year of life
8. Childhood morbidity
9. Childhood malignancy

*Modified from reference 8. Categories are not mutually exclusive.

reliability because of difficulty remembering when contraception was stopped or because of intermittent use of contraceptives. A third measure has also been suggested that consists of determining the number of living children among workers, then comparing that rate with age, parity, and race-specific numbers derived from the National Center for Health Statistics.[4] The limitations of this method are that it fails to control other important variables which help influence the number of children, such as socioeconomic status, and the fact that this method has not been validated in a large study that compares a traditional historical approach with this simplified methodology.

Pregnancy Loss

Fetal loss, a relatively common outcome, is often defined differently by different researchers. Several definitions are necessary to evaluate and compare studies using the rate of loss as an end point. First, one must define the gestation period: researchers generally use this term to refer to weeks since conception, while clinicians use it to denote weeks since the last menstrual period. Second, the time at which a woman may recognize a pregnancy must be defined, since improved diagnostic techniques and more widely available home use tests enable detection earlier than in the past. This is important, since recent work indicates that the rate of loss (sometimes early in pregnancy before a woman recognizes she is pregnant, but generally at six to eight weeks of gestation) may be as high as 75%.[5] These estimates are based on daily determinations of early pregnancy factor, a rosette inhibition test based on the production of a protein generally detectable within hours of conception in humans, or on determination of levels of human chorionic gonadotropin, which is secreted after implantation in the uterine wall. Much of this early fetal loss probably goes unrecognized unless one of these sensitive methods is used.

Many researchers use the terms spontaneous abortion and miscarriage to refer to early and late fetal loss, respectively, sometimes without specifying the temporal dividing line between the two. This problem is sometimes exacerbated by failure to say whether gestation is measured in weeks since last menstrual period or since estimated conception. Usually, spontaneous abortion refers to loss within 20 weeks of conception. Use of the term spontaneous fetal loss to refer to loss of a recognized pregnancy at any time avoids this confusion. There is little loss of precision with the inclusive term, since loss after 20 weeks is far less frequent than that which occurs earlier.

Most research to date has centered on early pregnancy loss (between 8 and 20 weeks of gestation). a number of excellent life tables accounting for the influencing variables of age, alcohol, smoking, and previous obstetrical history help to define the probability of fetal loss beyond the 8th week.[6,7] This information allows a rough estimate of "normal" or background rates of spontaneous fetal loss according to gestational age. The rate of fetal loss between the 8th and 20th weeks of gestation is approximately 15%. Of pregnancies which extend longer, the rate of spontaneous abortion is only about 2%. The study of a more rare outcome, such as late fetal loss, requires larger sample sizes than would be required for more common outcomes, but this need can be balanced against the improved reliability of diagnosis later in pregnancy.

Birth Defects

Among birth or developmental defects, the most studied is birth weight, probably because it is the easiest to ascertain. This index is routinely recorded on virtually all birth certificates in the United States. The incidence of low-birth-weight children (less than 2500 g) is approximately 7% in the United States. The incidence of major birth defects is approximately 3%. Ascertainment of major birth defects, however, depends on a number of important factors. First is the definition of what constitutes a major (as opposed to minor) birth defect. Generally, the definition which has been adopted is that of the Centers for Disease Control: those defects which affect survival, require substantial medical care, result in marked physical or psychological handicaps, or interfere with the baby's prospects for a productive, fulfilling life. A list exists of defects considered included in this definition.

Another important consideration is the length of follow-up for detection of birth defects, since less than half are detected before the child leaves the hospital. Thus, good ascertainment of birth defects requires follow-up and postnatal visits of the child. A third difficulty with studying the occurrence of major birth defects as an end point in reproductive studies is that no agent so far has been identified that increases the incidence of all defects. Thus one must study individual defects. The most common individual defects are neural tube defects, which constitute approximately 0.5% of live births in the United States. Severe mental retardation is lower at 0.4%, and chromosomal abnormality is 0.25%. One may also look at infant death or the incidence of death in the first year of life. The number of children who die during this period is approximately 2% of live births. Finally, recent attention has been focused on the incidence of childhood cancer. This is a rare outcome, with only a small number of investigations to date.

Sperm Evaluation

A promising approach to evaluation of one aspect of reproductive impairments is sperm evaluation. Sperm has been demonstrated to be a sensitive indicator of chemicals that affect sperm production, and studies of sperm have very modest sample size requirements.[8] Sperm is also easily obtainable, objectively evaluated, and a sensitive indicator of exposures of the previous 74 days (the spermatogenic period), and there are no female factors to consider. Parameters that can be studied among sperm include volume, concentration, motility, and morphology. Of these parameters, morphology seems most promising. The proportion of sperm with abnormal morphology has a low degree of variability, which means that the sample size required for a study is very modest. For example, a study of sperm morphology to reliably detect a 20% or greater change requires 52 men, half of which are exposed and half unexposed. A similar study of sperm concentration needs 428 men divided similarly between exposed and unexposed groups. This relationship seems to be independent of other factors that influence counts, such as abstinence period and recent fever.

Separate lines of evidence link abnormal sperm morphology and decreased concentrations to infertility and, with less certainty, to increased occurrence of fetal loss.[9] The count is difficult to use, since it has a large variability from one day to the next in an individual man. Motility is difficult because of problems in objectively evaluating it and its high sensitivity to the temperature and to the duration of the time between when it is collected and when it is examined.

AGENTS WITH KNOWN OR SUSPECTED TOXICITY

Chemicals with recognized reproductive toxicity in humans are summarized in Table 8-2, including the main occupational groups at risk and the specific associated abnormalities. This table also includes agents that have not been studied in human populations but that may have adverse effects in humans as judged by their adverse effects in animals. This table is notable in that a small number of agents are considered toxic relative to the large number of agents found in the working environment and that the majority of effects noted are found among women. The studies cited here are summarized from more extensive reviews that the reader may wish to consult.[10–12]

Table 8-2 summarizes the relatively few studies that have identified agents with chemical toxicity on reproduction. These studies nevertheless represent approximately 50% of all studies, so about half of all studies failed to demonstrate an association. The high proportion showing no association and the large number of chemicals in use lead one to suspect the existence of unrecognized toxicity. The methodological and logistic problems inherent in such work make it likely that fewer studies will be conducted in the future, and those that are will have more difficulty demonstrating an effect

Table 8-2
Agents with Reproductive Toxicity in Man or Animal

Agent	Uses or potential exposures	Reproductive effects: Humans, Males	Reproductive effects: Humans, Females	Reproductive effects: Animals (but no human evidence), Males	Reproductive effects: Animals (but no human evidence), Females
Anesthetic gases (including halothane)	Hospital operating room; dental clinics; veterinary surgeries	Impaired fertility	Impaired fertility, spontaneous abortion		
Arsenic	Manufacture of copper, lead, or alloys; glass insecticides or fungicides		Menstrual disorders, spontaneous abortion		
Benzo[a]pyrene	Reagent for determination of cadmium			Testicular damage, impaired fertility	Estrus cycle disorders
Benzene	Manufacture of chemicals, dyes, or other organic compounds; artificial leather, varnishes, lacquers; solvents		Abortion, spontaneous impaired fertility, menstrual disorders	Testicular damage	

Beryllium	Aerospace fabrications		Maternal death		
Boron	Weatherproofing, preservative, cosmetics		Impaired fertility		
Cadmium	Plating, photo-electric cells, dentistry				
Carbon monoxide	Persons exposed to automobile fumes		Low birth weight		
Chloroform	Solvent for oils, fats, resins, rubber		Impaired fertility		Fetotoxic
Chloroprene	Rubber manufacturers	Decreased libido, impotence			Fetotoxic
Dichloromethane	Degreasers and cleaners				
Epichlorohydrin	Solvent for resins, gums, paints, varnishes, lacquers			Reduced fertility	Testicular damage
Ethylene dibromide	Fruit fumigators; gasoline fumes				
Ethylene dichloride	Solvent for rubber, fats, oil, extract for tobacco				Fetotoxic

Table 8-2 (continued)

Agent	Uses or potential exposures	Reproductive effects			
		Humans		*Animals (but no human evidence)*	
		Males	Females	Males	Females
Ethylene oxide	Fumigant, sterilizing agents for surgical instruments, fungicide		Menstrual disorders, low weight	Spontaneous abortion	
Formaldehyde	Resins, leather, rubber, metals or wood; workers in pathology laboratories			Menstrual disorders, spontaneous abortion, low birth weight	
Hormones (androgens, estrogens, progestogens, synthetic hormones)	Pharmaceutical workers or researchers				
Lead	Automobile or aircraft exhaust fumes	Decreased libido		Spontaneous impotence, testicular damage or infertility	Abortion

Manganese	Manufacture of steel, glass, ink, dry cell batteries, ceramics, paint, rubber, welding rods, wood preservatives	Decreased libido		Impotence	
Mercury		Decreased libido, impotence	Low birth weight		Fetotoxic and embryo
Pesticides (including carbaryl, dibromochloropropane, kepone, malathion, 2,4,5-T)	Insecticides	Testicular damage or infertility			
Polybrominated biphenyls (PBBS)	Fire retardant in plastics, wood preservatives, electrical insulations			Impaired fertility	Fetotoxic
Polychlorinated biphenyls (PCBs)	Insulating materials in transformers and capacitators; hydraulic fluid		Menstrual disorders		

Table 8-2 (continued)

Agent	Uses or potential exposures	Reproductive effects			
		Humans		*Animals (but no human evidence)*	
		Males	Females	Males	Females
Selenium	Photography, electronic components instruments, rubber manufacture				Fetotoxic
Styrene	Manufacture of plastics, synthetic rubber, resins, insulators		Menstrual disorders		
Toluene	Benzoic acid, benzaldehyde, explosives, dye	Decreased libido, impotence	Menstrual disorder, low birth weight		
Vinyl chloride	Vinyl chloride, polyvinyl chloride, related products	Decreased libido, impotence	Low birth weight		
Xylene	Solvent				Fetotoxic

even if one exists. Included are problems with measuring exposure levels, dubious reliability of occupational histories and of ascertaining reproductive outcomes, bias that may be introduced by the presence of other influencing variables such as smoking and alcohol whose effects may overshadow those of the agent being studied, and difficulties obtaining a sample size adequate to demonstrate reliably subtle effects. These limitations are dealt with in greater detail in the "Challenges for Future Studies" portion of this chapter.

RESEARCH TO DATE

Observational Epidemiology

To date, approaches to defining agents that impair reproduction have followed three lines.[1] The first is observational epidemiology, which refers to the observations of astute clinicians or individual workers. Perhaps the most striking example of this comes from workers involved in a California plant who noted that all the men working in a certain portion of the plant seemed unable to produce children. Subsequent sperm analyses revealed marked abnormalities and led to the identification of DBCP as a potent inhibitor of spermatogenesis.

Toxicology

A second method of identifying reproductive problems associated with agents is toxicity. The toxicologist's story is one of mixed success and failure. For example, toxicology identified DBCP as a problem long before it came to clinical attention. Only after the emergence of a clinical problem associated with DBCP did review of the literature indicate that toxicologists had previously identified this risk. There are, on the other hand, also stories of success: toxicologists first identified waste anesthetic gases as causing reproductive problems in animals, and subsequent clinical studies confirmed the association between anesthetic gases and impaired fecundability and fetal loss in humans. To date, there has been no systematic review of the toxicology literature to ascertain the number and type of workers exposed to various agents in an attempt to set priorities for epidemiologic investigation.

Surveillance

Finally, the third approach is that of surveillance. Surveillance is defined as "the continued watchfulness over the distribution and trends of incidence through the systematic collection, consolidation, and evaluation of morbidity and mortality reports and other relevant data."[13] The most notable example of a surveillance system is that established by the United States and other countries around the world following the thalidomide trouble. The advantages of reproductive surveillance are that it provides background rates to define the risks in subpopulations, which may be a measure of consistency needed to judge the degree of risk, and also helps in evaluating clusters of problems. An example has emerged from the use of video display terminals, which has been raised as a possible cause of spontaneous abortion. This issue has been difficult to evaluate in part because of the lack of available information on women using video display terminals and their rates of reproductive loss. The second advantage of reproductive surveillance is that trends can be monitored. An example is that the Centers for Disease Control Birth Defects Monitoring program has revealed a steady decline in the incidence of neural tube defects in this country, with the exception of an increasing rate in Appalachia. A similar trend, but this time of increasing rates, has been observed for patent ductus arteriosus and ventriculoseptal defects. Both of these congenital malformations have been increasing. With both trends, however, the reasons behind the changes are unknown.

This points out the third advantage of reproductive surveillance, namely, that hypotheses and research priorities are generated. The fourth advantage is that surveillance may identify additional associations for recognized hazards. An example comes from a registry for angiosarcoma after this rare liver tumor was found to be associated with vinyl chloride. In subsequent case collection, a connection with a new agent, androgenic anabolic steroids, was discovered. The fifth advantage is that certain events may be more sensitive indicators of reproductive risks than others. For example, since it is more frequent, spontaneous abortion has been suggested as being a more sensitive indicator than live births of the risks of chromosomal abnormality. Sixth, reproductive surveillance provides a pool of control subjects, permitting their use as a comparison group for certain studies. The seventh and perhaps the most important role of the surveillance system is to provide reassurance about the lack of problems. Such an example comes from the birth defects monitoring programs around the world that have largely, since their inception, been reassuring about the lack of new problems.

AN EXAMPLE: INVESTIGATION OF REPRODUCTIVE PROBLEMS ASSOCIATED WITH VIDEO DISPLAY TERMINALS

The introduction and widespread adoption in the United States of video display terminals (VDT) has resulted in much interest in the safety of these devices. Particular attention has focused on possible adverse reproductive consequences. This concern has resulted in numerous inquiries about whether these machines are safe for men or women anticipating conception or for women who may be or are known to be pregnant. The following episode illustrates how such questions raised by an individual progressed through a corporate physician and culminated in a formal epidemiologic investigation.

An employee who worked in a large office building approached the consultant physician and expressed concern about a high number of recent problem pregnancies among her coworkers: many of the women had spontaneous abortions, and several of those who had carried the pregnancy to term had children with severe birth defects. All of those women worked with VDTs in the word processing division, and the employee was concerned about the safety of VDTs.

The physician began his investigation by asking the women in the word processing department whether they had been pregnant during the preceding year and what the outcome of the pregnancy was. Ten women reported becoming pregnant. Of these, six pregnancies ended in spontaneous fetal loss, three in children with congenital malformations, and only one in a normal, full-term delivery; there were no induced abortions. That nine of ten pregnancies should end atypically is clearly abnormal, and the physician called public health officials for assistance in investigating the possible connection between VDTs and these birth abnormalities.

What was intuitively clear in this instance to both the worker and the physician was that the number of problems that occurred was higher than expected. The epidemiologist who continued the investigation began by quantifying statistically how abnormal these events were. This procedure would be particularly useful when the presence of abnormalities is not clear. About 15% of recognized pregnancies end in spontaneous fetal loss, and approximately 3% of liveborn infants have a major congenital malformation (see "Assessing Reproductive Impairments"). Thus the probability that six or more of ten pregnancies will end in spontaneous fetal loss (calculated according to the binomial distribution) is 0.0013. Similarly, the probability that three or more of four children will be born with a major congenital malformation is 0.0001. That the physician observed 0.6 of the pregnancies ending in spontaneous fetal loss and 0.75 of the live births with congenital malformations clearly confirms the physician's perception of an abnormal event.

The epidemiologist continued the investigation by establishing standard definitions, confirming the number of reported events (the denominator), establishing the number of pregnancies (the numerator), and gaining background information on potential risk factors at the work site and information from each woman on factors that might influence the probability of pregnancy problems. A pregnancy was identified by a positive pregnancy test from a medical laboratory, a spontaneous abortion by a physician's diagnosis or a history that on medical review was most consistent with fetal loss, and a major congenital malformation by the definition presented earlier in "Assessing Reproductive Impairments." Employment records were reviewed, and all women who had worked in the word processing department during the previous year, including those who had since left the department or the company, were administered a comprehensive questionnaire that included previous medical and obstetrical history, use of drugs (including smoking and alcohol), VDT exposure, and other factors considered possibly relevant. At the time these interviews were being conducted, the work site was examined and, with the help of industrial hygienists, any materials that might present a risk of fetal loss or congenital problems were noted.

The researcher confirmed the occurrence of each reported episode of fetal loss or congenital malformation (such episodes are frequently overreported, particularly in such an emotional situation, and need confirmation) and also discovered five additional pregnancies. Of those pregnancies, two were terminated by spontaneous fetal loss and three by the delivery of full-term, healthy infants. Physically, the work site was a portion of a large office building that was 15 years old and, apart from regular spraying of insecticides, had no suspicious exposures. Investigation of the agents used to spray insects began with determining which agents were used. The product safety sheets for each (available from the manufacturer) were then reviewed and a library search done utilizing MEDLINE and TOXLINE for background literature on reproductive risk.

Although this research revealed that the agents could cause spontaneous fetal loss in animals, such events were limited to high dosages, which the researcher felt were unlikely to be present in the office building. An extensive review of the literature on VDTs revealed no studies of reproduction in humans but a modest literature on the radiation produced by such machines and the risks associated with various kinds and levels of radiation in animals.

At this point, a picture emerged that was clearly abnormal. Realizing that a comparison group would be necessary to evaluate the risk of VDTs, the researcher identified a group of women office workers from another portion of the same building who did not work with VDTs. This group was interviewed in the same manner as the women working with VDTs and administered the same questionnaire. After reviewing the responses, the epidemiologist arranged his findings as shown in Table 8-3.

Among the group using VDTs, the risk of spontaneous fetal loss was 3.2 (95% confidence interval, 1.0–10.5) times higher and congenital malformations 2.3 (0.3–19.8) times higher than in the nonexposed group.

The epidemiologist now found himself in a quandary: the information was consistent with an association with VDTs, but the number of events was too small to provide statistical reliability, and the background literature failed to reveal a biologic basis that would make such an association credible. His next step, therefore, was to look more closely at the relationship between degree of exposure to VDTs and the likelihood of spontaneous abortion (dose–response relationship). Congenital malformations were too few to be able to compare the rates among exposed women according to degree of exposure. The number of women with spontaneous fetal loss was too small to divide into more than two broad subgroups of workers according to the number of hours per day they spent on the machine, the total number of hours worked during the first trimester of pregnancy, and the proximity of the

Table 8-3
Exposure to Video Display Terminals

	Spontaneous fetal loss		Total pregnancies	Relative risk	95% Confidence interval
	Yes	*No*			
Exposure to VDTs					
Yes	8	7	15	3.2	1.0–10.5
No	2	10	12		
	Congenital Malformation				
	Yes	*No*	Total live births		
Exposure to VDTs					
Yes	3	4	7	2.3	0.3–19.8
No	1	7	8		

machines to each woman's work station. These investigations found that the problems were no more frequent in the women with higher degrees of exposure. This absence of dose–response relationship detracts from the likelihood of association between VDT exposure and the reproductive problems studied.

In trying to reconcile the overall suggestion of an association with the absence of dose–response relationship, the researcher thought again about the likelihood of biologically significant amounts of radiation that might be produced by the machines. The literature review indicated that most VDTs, and particularly the newer machines, tended to be well below the levels at which biological effects might be produced. Because the machines in this office might have been emitting more radiation than they should have, he asked the industrial hygienists to measure the radiation. Those levels were below the limits of detection and thus well below levels that might be biologically active.

The researcher concluded that although there was a suspicious overall association of these abnormal reproductive events with VDTs, such an association was biologically implausible (as supported by the lack of a relationship between more frequent adverse events in women who were most heavily exposed). In the absence of definitive evidence, he recommended instituting a surveillance program to monitor women who became pregnant.

During the next year and a half, 14 women became pregnant. All 14 pregnancies resulted in healthy, full-term deliveries. The company, the consulting physician, and the epidemiologist concluded that there appeared to be no association between VDTs and reproductive problems and that the earlier problems most likely represented a statistical quirk. To be certain, however, the surveillance program was continued.

This episode and its investigation illustrate several points. First, clinicians are frequently presented with unfamiliar problems involving exposures that may be unknown. Most frequently, the questions involve an individual or small group, which does not provide a large enough sample for a statistically reliable study drawing clear conclusions about the presence of reproductive risk. In these circumstances, the clinician can draw on the available literature and, of course, request the assistance of public health officials. The National Institute for Occupational Safety and Health has a program designed specifically to provide assistance in such occupational questions. Its parent organization, the Centers for Disease Control, has a similar program that deals more broadly with issues of public health concern. Second, and similarly a limitation of the small number of people in this example, is the difficulty in drawing clear conclusions in the face of few previous studies. This difficulty is exemplified by the task this epidemiologist faced in making recommendations about actions to protect employees' health. This also demonstrated that even though statistically certain events are highly improbable, they do occur. In the context of spontaneous fetal loss, one may consider that the probability of any five pregnancies all terminating in spontaneous fetal loss is $(0.15)^6 = 0.0001$, or 1/10,000, but given the likelihood of there being 10,000 groups of five women working with VDTs who become pregnant, the probability of at least one such group of five is 0.63. Perhaps most importantly, however, this event demonstrates the need for further investigation to define the magnitude of reproductive problems associated with VDTs in order to take preventive measures or else to provide reassurance about the absence of such a problem.

CHALLENGES FOR FUTURE STUDIES

One of the most important considerations in deciding what outcome to study is the number of events (such as episodes of fetal loss or other end points) required for a study. Several of the outcomes from Table 8-1 are included in Table

Table 8-4
Sample Size Required to Detect Twofold Increase in Adverse Reproductive Outcomes*

Outcome	Background rate (%)	Sample Size†
Fecundability		
Infertility	10	436 couple-years
Pregnancy loss		
≤20 weeks' gestation	15	322 pregnancies
21+ weeks' gestation	2	1856 pregnancies
Birth/developmental defects		
Low birth weight	7	586 live births
Major birth defects (all)	3	1262 live births
Neural tube defect	1	3638 live births
Infant death (≤1 year)	2	1856 live births

*Modified from reference 8. $\alpha = 0.05$, $\beta = 0.20$.
†Divided evenly between exposed and unexposed groups.

8-4, along with the sample sizes required to reliably detect a doubling in incidence. The effect of these large sample requirements is to make studies logistically difficult.

One may take these sample size requirements a step further by considering the population size of working persons required to do a study. For example, given that the fertility rate in working women is 44 per 1000 women per year, and the spontaneous abortion rate is 15 per 100 pregnancies, then the pregnancy rate in working women is equal to 52 per 1000 women per year (44 ÷ 0.85). To perform a study of spontaneous abortion in this population, 322 pregnancies are needed. To observe this number of pregnancies in a year, the number of women equals the number of pregnancies divided by the pregnancy rate, or 6220 women (322 ÷ 52 per 1000). If the unreasonably optimistic assumption is made that each woman has been exposed an average of five years, the number of women would decrease by a factor of 5, or 1244 women (6220 ÷ 5). We need then to consider that working women represent 43% of the labor force, so we would need an occupational population of nearly 3000 persons (1244 ÷ 0.43). The problem becomes even more complex when one considers the difficulty of finding a stable population. Occupational exposures are nearly always multiple; working with only a single agent is quite rare. Separating the effect of a single exposure of interest from multiple exposures, including such nonoccupational exposures as smoking and alcohol, requires larger samples.

Other difficulties include reliability of ascertaining exposure and outcome indices. Many exposures are difficult to characterize, in regard to either quantity or content. Keeping track of exposures to individual agents is generally difficult, inconvenient, and may be uncomfortable or dangerous for the worker. Sampling is generally not done for agents without clearly demonstrated toxicity, so records are generally unsuitable for investigation of new relationships. The reproductive outcomes that research generally seeks to identify are relatively rare, and the degree of impairment is often subtle. For example, one of the most frequently studied outcomes is spontaneous abortion, which occurs in only 15% of recognized pregnancies. The occurrence of neural tube defects is less than 1%. Finally, the effects of occupational exposures are probably quite small when compared to the effects of common exposures such as smoking and alcohol.

The need for large populations also poses other problems of where studies can be conducted. Reproductive research tends to be centered in large companies that provide an adequate number of workers for study and the possibility of an unexposed group for comparison (control group). These larger companies are under greater scrutiny and are more likely to be able to afford protective measures, to employ industrial hygienists, and to spend money to assure protection. Smaller shops that may be struggling for their financial survival and that employ small numbers are the places where problems are more likely to occur.

CONCLUSIONS

Despite recent interest in the relationship between the working environment and reproduction, only a handful of the many thousands of chemical, biological, and physical agents have been examined for their reproductive effects in humans. While toxicology helps provide clues about reproductive toxicity and helps the clinician indirectly in assessing possible occupational contribution to reproductive impairments, the dearth of information generally means that clinicians must make clinical decisions based on incomplete or nonexistent information.

A host of methodological problems accompanies studies of occupation and reproduction, the foremost of which is the need for a large, stable occupational group. Although few studies are capable of surmounting most of these problems, the observations of astute clinicians have been central to identifying occupational agents that history indicates are clearly capable of impairing reproduction. Although the magnitude of toxic effect cannot be estimated at present, the large number of working men and women and the very large number of agents used in the work environment suggest the possibility of unrecognized toxicity.

REFERENCES

1. Rosenberg MJ, Halperin WE: The role of surveillance in monitoring reproductive health. *Teratogenisis Carcinog Mutagen* 1984; 4:15–24.
2. Rosenstock L: Occupational medicine: Too long neglected. *Ann Intern Med* 1981;95:774–776.
3. National Center for Health Statistics, Mosher CVD, Pratt WF: *Reproductive Impairments Among Married Couples: United States.* Washington, US Government Printing Office, December, 1962.
4. Levine RJ, Symons MJ, Balogh SA, et al: A method for monitoring the fertility of workers. I. Method and pilot studies. *J Occup Med* 1980;22:781–791.

5. Roberts CJ, Lowe CR: Where have all the conceptions gone? *Lancet* 1983;1:498–499.
6. Harlap S, Shiono PH, Ramcharan S: A Life Table of Spontaneous Abortions and the Effects of Age, Parity, and Other Variables, in Hook EB, Porter I (eds): *Reproductive Loss.* New York, Academic Press, 1981, p 81.
7. French FE, Bierman JM: Probabilities of fetal mortality. *Public Health Rep* 1962;77:10.
8. Wyrobek AJ, Gordon LA, Burkhart JC, et al: An evaluation of human sperm as indicators of chemically induced alterations of spermatogenic function: A report of the gene-tox program. *Mutat Res* 1983;115:73–148.
9. Rosenberg MJ, Wyrobek AJ, Ratcliffe J, et al: Sperm as an indicator of reproductive risk among petroleum refinery workers. *Br J Occup Med* 1985;42:123–127.
10. Bloom AD, (ed): *Guidelines for Studies of Human Populations Exposed To Mutagenic and Reproductive Hazards.* New York, March of Dimes Birth Defects Foundation, 1981.
11. Rosenberg MJ, Feldblum PJ, Marshall EG, et al: Epidemiologic surveillance of occupational effects on reproduction. Contract report to the US Office of Technology Assessment for *Assessment of Reproductive Hazards in the Workplace.* Washington, DC, US Government Printing Office, 1985.
12. Barlow SM, Sullivan FM: *Reproductive Hazards of Industrial Chemicals.* New York, Academic Press, 1982.
13. Langmuir AD: The surveillance of communicable diseases of natural importance. *N Engl J Med* 1963;182–192.

CHAPTER 9

INTERNATIONAL INFANT FORMULA CONTROVERSIES

Janine M. Jason, MD
Gene A. McGrady, MD

The prevalence of breast-feeding in the United States and in other nations has for many years been a subject of interest to health workers.[1,2] Since the 1960s and possibly earlier, there has been concern that the trend away from breast-feeding toward use of commercial preparations may have exacerbated the problems of protein malnutrition and diarrheal disease among infants in developing nations.[3–5] These sentiments began to be most vocally expressed in the early 1970s. The 1972 publication of an article entitled "Commerciogenic Malnutrition?"[6] heralded a movement which eventually resulted in the adoption by the World Health Organization (WHO) of the International Code of Marketing of Breast-Milk Substitutes.[7] On May 21, 1981, this code was adopted in the assembly of WHO by a vote of 118 countries in favor, three abstaining, and one opposing. The only opposing vote was cast by the representative of the United States. The US vote was made in the face of strongly conflicting viewpoints within this country and perhaps galvanized these conflicting factions further.

In this paper we will attempt to present an historical perspective on: (1) the levels and substance of the disagreements within the United States which preceded and affected the US vote, (2) how US representatives (among others), attempted to develop compromises for a final version of the code that might have permitted the United States to vote in the affirmative, and (3) briefly, some outcomes of the vote, the controversy, and the code itself. We will attempt the perhaps impossible task of being evenhanded in our presentations of differing viewpoints, but caution the readers to be circumspect about their own biases, as well as the author's. No attempt will be made to discuss the disagreements occurring on an international level that may have influenced or may have evolved from this issue. We will also not deal in depth with the scientific basis of differing viewpoints. While the latter is essential to judging the merits of some of the conflicts, the scientific issues have been reviewed extensively in at least one document,[8] which is recommended to the reader. We will, then, first briefly outline the code itself in its final form; second, present some of the legal, scientific, and emotional aspects of the published disagreements with the United States; third, present some of the United States' attempts at compromise versions of the code; fourth, present the ostensible reason for the vote itself; and last, attempt to provide some insight into the outcome of these disagreements and of the code itself.

The "International Code of Marketing of Breast-Milk Substitutes" applies to the marketing of infant formula, other milk products, and all other foods or beverages represented as possible replacements for breast milk. It recommends that information and education regarding infant feeding be a governmental responsibility directly or through regulation of any other agency providing such information. It specifies, furthermore, that all such educational or informational material should include the following points: (1) the benefits and superiority of breast-feeding; (2) the importance of maternal nutrition and maternal preparation for breast-feeding; (3) the negative effects of partial bottle feeding; (4) the difficulty of reversing the decision not to breast-feed; and (5) the proper use of infant formula.

Advertisement and other forms of promotion of breast-milk substitutes to the general public is prohibited by the code. The giving of product samples or other gifts in promotion of the use of breast-milk substitutes is likewise prohibited. Through the provisions of article 6, the code attempts to ensure that health care workers and health care facilities do not directly or indirectly promote use of infant formula except where medically indicated. It attempts also to protect employees of manufacturers and distributors of breast-milk substitutes from the negative effects of constraints on marketing practices by providing that bonuses and sales quotas should not apply to the products covered by the code. Clear and conspicuous labeling of breast-milk substitutes is required. Finally, the code states that governments are responsible for implementing the code and monitoring its effectiveness. The mechanisms appropriate to the implementation of the code are left for member countries to determine. The code also holds manufacturers and distributors directly responsible, independent of governmental measures, for monitoring their marketing practices. Governments of member states are required to communicate annually to the director-general of WHO on all actions taken to implement the principles and aims of the code.[7]

The US assistant secretary of state for international organization affairs stated that the reasons the United States could not support the code as outlined above rested on both legal and governmental grounds. First, there was concern that it might set a precedent for WHO filling a regulatory role over member nations, a role that the United States could not accept. Second, despite an opinion from the antitrust division of the Justice Department to the contrary, there was an expressed concern that if it were adopted in the United States it would violate First Amendment rights and antitrust laws.[9] The legal aspects of these disagreements reflected debates occurring during the formulation of the code itself about whether it should be regulatory or recommendatory in nature. As finally written, the code is recommendatory but requires that WHO be notified of violations.[7] In fact, WHO does not have any mechanism available for enforcement, and thus the code could not be regulatory in nature, unless it were made regulatory by a member country, through enactment by that country's governing body. The US government, however, remained concerned that it could not support an act which it felt it could not legally enforce at home, especially since the WHO resolution adopting the code encouraged its adoption by all member countries. While the legal issues themselves are not the topic of this paper, they do introduce three major sectors affected by the code and intimately involved in the controversies surrounding it, ie, business, health professionals, and the public.

Not surprisingly, American formula-makers felt the code would restrict their abilities to market to both the public and to health professionals and that is misrepresented as harmful the effects of partial, if not exclusive, formula-feeding. In 1978, a US Senate subcommittee hearing received testimony from representatives of several major infant formula manufacturers. In their view, the proposed code assumed an unproven relationship between the promotion and marketing of infant formula and the prevalence of breast-feeding in less developed countries (LDC). It was their opinion that the availability of manufactured breast milk did not affect the numbers of mothers breast-feeding. In general, the US companies agreed that the promotion of infant formula directly to the public was ethically improper. They felt, however, that promotion to health care workers could not be considered unethical behavior.[10] These firms accordingly attempted to influence the administration, health professionals, and the public against the code through intensive lobbying and publicity.[11,12] Grocery manufacturers and pharmaceutical companies also felt threatened by the code, fearing that it would set a precedent for future action restricting other business marketing practices and would give credence to critics of "big business." Therefore, representatives of these business interests joined formula-makers in their lobbying efforts.

The medical community was not unified in its response to the code on either an organizational or individual level. The American Academy of Pediatrics opposed the code; the Ambulatory Pediatric Association supported it. Other medical organizations resented not being included in the decision-making process of the United States until the final draft of the code had been made.[13] Individual medical opinions were similarly divided. The disagreements appeared to lie in four main areas. First, does scientific evidence support that there is a relationship between formula marketing practices and/or formula use and infant morbidity and mortality? Second, does the code address issues truly pertinent to infant morbidity and mortality? Third, is the code inflexible to the varying needs of different individuals, different situations, and different nations? Fourth, is making a statement concerning an important public health need more important than the actual details of that statement?

Editorials appearing in one issue of the journal *Pediatrics* give a sampling of the different points of view. One editorial, in opposition to the code, reasoned that the marketing practices for infant formula should be changed if, in fact, they lead to increasing infant morbidity and mortality. These practices might adversely affect morbidity and mortality if they contribute to a decline in the prevalence of breast-feeding in developing nations; however, no such cause–effect relation between marketing practices for infant formula and the prevalence of breast-feeding can be shown to exist. Other factors, including maternal employment and changing cultural attitudes, were largely responsible for the declining prevalence of breast-feeding in developing nations, and programs oriented toward these factors would be more effective than a code on marketing. Further, the author suggested that the controversy over the code had diverted efforts and resources from remedying undebatable causes of infant morbidity and mortality in impoverished regions, including unsanitary conditions, infection, malnutrition, lack of education, etc.[14]

Pediatricians who supported the code did not raise any different issues. One editorial in the same issue of *Pediatrics* referenced numerous studies of varying quality and quoted several experts supporting the contention that marketing practices do indeed decrease the prevalence of breast-feeding and lead to increased infant morbidity and mortality. Further, it noted that "the problems of infant morbidity and mortality will not be solved only by restricting the marketing of breast-milk substitutes. Poverty, lack of sanitation and clean water, illiteracy, malnutrition, harmful cultural practices, and unavailability of appropriate health care are all contributing factors. Massive social upheavals in some parts of the world have addressed these problems and made significant inroads against them. The need for social change should not, however, prevent approaches that can be adopted now and that have been demonstrated to produce partial solutions. Implementation of the WHO code is one such approach".[12]

In addition to the business and health care sectors, the third sector actively involved in the formula-marketing controversy included coalitions of individuals with strong opinions about the ethics of marketing practices in LDCs and about the effects of breast-milk substitutes on infant health in these countries. The most vocal and best organized of these groups included the Infant Formula Action Coalition (INFACT) and the Interfaith Center on Corporate Responsibility of the National Council of Churches. These groups initiated boycotts which were apparently economically effective against nonformula products manufactured by formula companies, in order to exert pressure upon these companies to change their marketing practices in LDCs. The significance of this sector's role in regard to the code is reflected in the fact that in October 1979, INFACT was invited to participate in an international WHO–UNICEF meeting, although they had no official governmental status.

In outlining the disagreements surrounding the US vote on the code in a logical fashion, it is important to emphasize the strong and perhaps inevitable emotional component to these debates. This emotional element surfaced repeatedly in arguments presented by all the concerned sectors and undoubtedly was a major impediment to compromise and resolution of the differing opinions outlined above. This emotionalism is evident in newspaper headlines from that period, ranging from "A Totalitarian Grab for Baby's Bottle"[15] to "Hail to Free Enterprise—and Let the Babies Pay."[16] It is similarly evident in the editorials from *Pediatrics* noted above, eg, in equating publicity techniques used by groups supporting the code to "the vile, unsupported accusations and insinuations Senator McCarthy used in the political witch-hunt for Communists in the 1950's"[14] or in the use of exclamatory phrases to defend the United States vote: "The final vote in the World Health Organization was 118 to 1. The United States was the one! Does that mean that the United States was wrong? No, it only means that we didn't join in the stampede to place the blame for a significant share of a country's high infant mortality on foreign formula companies' advertising practices."[16,17]

Having presented the nature of the disagreements concerning this issue, we will not attempt to outline the events within WHO that led up to the creation of and vote on the code. WHO first become involved with breast-feeding as a health issue in 1973, at a time when opinions within the United States had not yet crystallized into widely publicized confrontations. In that year it entered a collaboration to research the frequency and duration of breast-feeding in several different countries.[18] At the 1974 meeting of WHO, the representative of the United Kingdom introduced, as co-sponsor, a draft resolution on the subject of breast-feeding. In final form the resolution strongly recommended the encouragement of breast-feeding as the ideal feeding for infants, called attention to the necessity of taking adequate social measures for mothers working away from their homes during the lactation period (eg, arranging special work schedules enabling continuation of breast-feeding), urged member nations to review promotion and advertisement of baby foods and to introduce remedial measures such as advertisement codes, urged the director-general to actively promote breast-feeding through its agencies, and urged the director-general to promote and support activities related to the preparation and use of weaning foods based on local products.[19] This resolution was adopted and the representative of the United States neither recorded any objection to the proposed draft resolution nor offered amendments.

In October 1979, WHO and UNICEF held a joint meeting on infant feeding to consider, among other things, the appropriate marketing and distribution of breast-milk substitutes. Representatives of governments, of the infant food industry, and of other concerned parties attended the meeting. The recommendations from that joint meeting were as follows:[20]

1. The practice of breast-feeding should be encouraged and supported.
2. Appropriate weaning practices should be promoted and supported.
3. Education, training, and information regarding breast-feeding and appropriate weaning practices should be promoted.
4. The health and social status of women in relation to infant and young child feeding should be promoted.
5. The appropriate marketing and distribution of breast-milk substitutes should be promoted through the establishment of an international code of marketing of infant formula and other products used as breast-milk substitutes.

The Thirty-Third World Health Assembly meeting in May 1980 endorsed these recommendations over the objections of the US delegation. This marked the beginning of a prolonged attempt by the United States to initiate compromises to WHO recommendations regarding breast-feeding. For reference, parts of the resolution appear below and amendments offered by the US delegation are included where they differ from the official version.

4. To prepare an international code of marketing of breast-milk substitutes in close consultation with member states and with all other parties concerned including such scientific and other experts whose collaboration may be deemed appropriate.[20]

4′. To prepare an international code of marketing of breast-milk substitutes *by convening a working group of all interested member states,* and by consulting with all other parties concerned including such scientific and other experts whose collaboration may be deemed appropriate.[21]

5. To submit the code to the executive board for consideration at its sixty-seventh session and for forwarding with its recommendations to the Thirty-Fourth World Health Assembly, together with proposals regarding its promotion and implementation, either as a regulation in the sense of articles 21 and 22 of the Constitution of the World Health Organization or as a recommendation in the sense of article 23, outlining the legal and other implications of each choice.[21]

The draft resolution had been discussed and debated through four meetings of the group responsible for its writing, a group which included a US representative. A consensus had been reached through those meetings; however, prior to the vote, the United States proposed the amendments appearing in the primed and italicized version above.

The US representative explained that the intent of the amendments was to explicitly and clearly provide a role to be played by governments of member states in preparing the draft code, because the US government had been concerned with the mechanism proposed for the elaboration of this international code. It did not want this type of mechanism to become a precedent.[20] The amendments were voted down, and the draft resolution adopted.

The draft code was submitted to the executive board session meeting in January 1981. The representative of the United States raised two objections to the proposed code at that meeting. First, he noted that the US government would strongly object if the code were adopted as a regulation, rather than a recommendation. Second, the US government had reservations on the content of the code. He specifically mentioned that the complete ban on advertisement to the public, provided for by the code, was a matter of serious concern.[22] The executive board approved the draft resolution and forwarded it to the Thirty-Fourth World Health Assembly, recommending its adoption.

In May 1981 the code was first considered by committee. The US representative again noted his nation's opposition to enactment of the code. He explained that the US government felt that the positive aspects of the code, ie, the promotion and protection of breast-feeding, were not sufficient to overcome its negative aspects, ie, a rigid set of rules applicable to companies, health workers, and health care systems throughout the world and provisions which would cause serious legal and constitutional problems for the United States. He again expressed the United States' concern about the World Health Organization's involvement in commercial codes, stating that this involvement was a central basis for the United States' inability to support the code.[23]

The proposed code was voted out of committee, 93 in favor, three opposed, and nine abstaining. The entire assembly next considered the code and adopted it. The United States was the only member state to maintain this opposition on the final vote. Throughout its opposition to the code, the US government consistently expressed the opinion that the WHO should not assume for itself the task of establishing and promoting international codes. Such tasks were seen as the responsibility of states.

Following adoption of the International Code of Marketing of Breast-Milk Substitutes, the United States commissioned two studies to be done. One commission was to examine the scientific evidence regarding the relation of breast-feeding to infant health; the other was to examine what should be done within the United States in response to the code. The first has been completed and was recently published.[8] That study was divided into a domestic and an international portion. The executive summary of that report concludes that domestically "breast-feeding does appear to decrease an infant's risk of gastrointestinal infection and otitis media. The effect of method of infant feeding on risk of other infections and allergies is less certain." The executive summary of the international portion states that "rates of gastrointestinal illnesses are lower among breast-fed infants and when such illness is an important cause of death, infant mortality from this cause appears to be reduced . . . Evidence of the effect of breast-feeding on respiratory tract and other infections from other studies was less clear."

Since the summary emphasizes the role of infectious diseases in infant morbidity and mortality associated with infant-feeding practices in developing countries, we will review here the intent and the conclusions of the chapter concerning that topic in some detail.[24] In that chapter, the authors attempted to determine whether method of infant feeding (breast vs other) was associated with: (1) differences in rates of infant mortality due to infectious, noninfectious, and all causes in LDCs; (2) differences in rates of infectious morbidity in LDCs; (3) differences in rates of infection due to specific pathogens; (4) differences in rates of infection specific to various organ systems; (5) and differences in morbidity and mortality in high-risk infants. In assessing various studies they applied criteria traditionally considered evidence of a causal association in classic epidemiologic studies. First, did the study take into account factors that may be associated with both making the decision about feeding method and with the outcome being assessed (eg, low socioeconomic status and infant mortality)? The methods used to do this could vary, but dealing with this problem in some manner was essential. Indeed, authors used a variety of techniques to deal with these issues, but the majority of authors did not deal with them at all.

Two studies dealt quite well with these criteria. The first was a study by Narayanan et al.[25] This study was performed in New Delhi, India, and included 261 low-birth-weight infants in a neonatal special care unit. The study was limited to infants fed at the time of admission and who remained in the nursery for at least three days. Comparison groups were matched for the presence of prolonged labor, premature rupture of membranes, maternal infection, daily exams, asphyxia, and birth weights. A randomized block design was used in the first year of the study; in the second year of the study the maximum number possible were fed human milk (all human milk was manually expressed). Cultures were performed on both (an unknown number of) formula samples (all samples negative for pathogens) and on 454 human milk samples. Sixty-five per cent of the milk samples were negative, 22% grew nonpathogenic organisms, and 13% grew potential pathogens; however, only one infant receiving culture-positive milk developed infection, and the organisms involved in this infection differed from that growing in the milk culture.

The investigators divided their population into four groups, matched as described above. These groups included the following: group 1, fed raw human milk between 9:00 AM and 9:00 PM and Holder-pasteurized human milk between 9:00 PM and 9:00 AM; group 2, fed raw human milk between 9:00 AM and 9:00 PM and nursery formula between 9:00 PM and 9:00 AM; group 3, colostrum (obtained ≤ 72 h after delivery) three times a day to a maximum of 20 cc every feeding, supplemented with nursery formula; and group 4, nursery formula only. Narayanan et al reaffirmed the quality of their matching by determining that all groups were similar in regard to matching criteria, including birth weight, gestational age, and matching risk factors. Groups 1–3 had fewer infections than Group 4 ($P < 0.001$), and there were no major infections in group 1. For those not having infections, the mean nursery stay was longer for groups 1–3, secondary to a longer survival of the premature infants in those groups (group 1 vs group 4, $P < 0.05$). For those having infection the mean stay was longer for group 4 (vs group 2, $P < 0.05$).

A second study, published by Butz et al in 1984, dealt with the issue of potential confounding factors in a more sophisticated way, in a less controlled environment.[26] These authors evaluated 52 primary sampling units (49 random) in peninsular Malaysia as part of the 1976–1977 Malaysia Family Life Survey. This survey included a three-round field survey of private households with one or more ever-married women less than 50 years of age. The total number of households was 1262; the total number of live singleton births was 5573. Infant deaths totaled 270 (4.8% of births). Women were asked to complete a "female retrospective life history" questionnaire which included questions concerning duration of supplemented/unsupplemented breast-feeding. A life-table approach, using a linear probability model estimated by ordinary least squares, was used. Variables included whether households had toilets and/or piped water. The authors concluded that:

(1) unsupplemented and supplemented breast-feeding are important for infant survival in homes without piped water and toilet sanitation; (2) unsupplemented breast-feeding is important at 8–28 days even with modern sanitation, supplemented breast-feeding makes little difference; (3) modern sanitation is more beneficial in areas where women breast-feed little or none.

A second criteria used to evaluate studies of infant morbidity and mortality in LDCs concerned the presence or absence of a demonstrated dose–response effect. Two studies provide reasonably good examples of the few studies meeting this criteria. Clavano evaluated 9622 infants delivered at a large hospital in the Philippines between January 1973 and April 1977.[27] Changes in feeding and in rooming policies occurred in the hospital during that time period. Although these must be considered in evaluating this study, one finding of note was that diarrheal illness rates among infants receiving breast-feeding, mixed feeding, and bottle feeding for the entire period studied were 0.9/1000, 13/1000, and 48/1000, respectively. Rates of mortality from ill-defined "clinical sepsis" among infants in these three groups were 0.03%, 0.16%, and 2.46%, respectively.

In another study, Kanaaneh retrospectively evaluated 610 healthy, full-term children aged 6–30 months, seen at Maternal and Child Health Stations in three Arabic villages in Israel.[28] The author looked at infant hospitalization in the first six months of life, broken down by that infant's feeding experience in the first six months of life. Rates of hospitalization were 0.5% for those breast-fed only, 2.9% for those breast-fed for greater than three but less than six months, 7.0% for those given mixed feedings for greater than three months, and 24.8% for those bottle fed only for greater than three months. These trends were mirrored in the rate of hospitalization for gastrointestinal illness in the first six months of life. It might be noted here, however, that this study did not meet the first criterion discussed above in an adequate manner, ie, the author did not apparently deal with potentially confounding factors.

The third question asked in the review was how strong was the association between feeding mode and the outcome studied? In the Kanaaneh study discussed above,[28] the relative risk of diarrheal illness was nearly 50 times greater for infants exclusively bottled fed compared with infants who were exclusively breast-fed, in the same Arab village. A separate study by Glass et al in 1983 provides a more elegant example of one meeting this criteria.[29] This study evaluated a well-defined surveillance area in Bangladesh between September 1980 and August 1981. Index cases of cholera were identified at Matlab Hospital and families of culture-confirmed cholera patients were recruited within 24 h of the index case's admission. Mothers were included when they did not have diarrhea in the previous week and had an infant less than 30 months old. The families received 10 daily home visits, and the study excluded those who were not present for at least four of those visits. The study included 93 mother–infant pairs. The researchers evaluated cholera antibodies in breast milk to the O-antigenic lypopolysaccharide of the outer membrane of *V. cholerae* 01 (high levels ≥ 250 units/mg IgA) and to cholera toxin (high levels ≥ 6 units/mg IgA). These titers are known to not be correlated with one another, but these antibodies are known to act synergistically in animals to protect against challenge with the *V. cholerae* 01. Daily stool samples were obtained for *V. cholerae* 01, and the mothers were questioned concerning diarrheal symptoms in the children. Clinical cholera was defined as ≥3 watery stools a day or ≥4 loose stools a day, within 24 h of a cholera-positive stool culture. Blood and breast-milk samples were obtained on day one of the study.

Thirty infants were found to be colonized after day one, and 19 of these infants had diarrhea. Breast-milk antibody levels were not correlated to colonization but, among the colonized, breast-milk antibody levels were correlated with symptoms. Children who drank breast milk with high vs low levels of antibodies were compared with the following results: for anti-cholera toxin, those with high levels were 60% as likely to have diarrhea as those with low levels ($P = 0.093$, Fisher's exact test (FET); for anti-lipopolysaccharide antibody, 51% as likely to have diarrhea ($P = 0.02$ FET); and for anti-cholera toxin × anti-lipopolysaccharide antibody, 40% as likely to have diarrhea ($P = 0.005$ FET). The authors had similar findings when they did not adjust for total IgA levels. They found no correlation with the mothers' serum total IgA or serum vibriocidal antitoxin titers and found no correlation between symptoms and total breast-milk IgA.

The final criterion raised in this review was, when full information was not given or obtained in a study and/or when possible biases or study weaknesses were not controlled for, in what direction would these lacks or biases affect the author's results? This criterion was, unfortunately, an important one to be used in most of the studies reviewed. Very often, however, the directions of these biases would have minimized or decreased the strength of the author's results. For example, if, in a given study, infants receiving mixed feedings were included in either the exclusively breast-fed group or the exclusively bottle-fed groups, this would lessen the likelihood of finding a difference between breast-fed and artificially fed infants. This type of grouping was frequently done. Thus, any difference found might be expected to have been stronger if biases or related factors had been considered in the analysis.

Using the above criteria, the authors reviewing the role of feeding mode on infectious disease morbidity and mortality in LDCs concluded that the literature supported an association between method of infant feeding and infectious diseases in LDCs. However, the review also supported that other factors, eg, sanitation and water source, may be as important or more important than feeding mode in regard to infant mortality in LDCs. Specifically, the authors felt that the evidence was strongest for an association between (1) feeding mode and overall infant mortality and (2) feeding mode and diarrheal illness. The literature also strongly supported that breast milk protects the high-risk newborn and that this protection was a direct effect and not due to the infant's avoidance of contaminated food substances. The literature was not conclusive concerning the areas of overall infant morbidity, respiratory infection, and allergic illness.

A second commission was asked to examine what needed to be done within the United States in response to the code.[30] This report concluded that breast-feeding in the United States has been increasing since the 1970s, and education concerning the support of breast feeding is available to the American woman from a variety of sources. US medical and federal agencies, including the Department of Health and Human Services, provide information and consultation concerning breast-feeding and nutrition to providers of primary health care, as well as to the general public. This report also noted that employment of working mothers was facilitated by the Pregnancy Discrimination Act adopted in 1978 and that government and private-sector initiatives provide day care services, food subsidies, and tax credits to full-time students and working parents. The report further noted that although the aims and principals of the international code are supported by both the "public and private sectors in the United States, some of the specific approaches to marketing practices for breast-milk substitutes set forth in the code are already in effect in the United States as a result of voluntary decisions by the major infant formula companies." Further, it noted that "the US government has reviewed the code and, as a general matter, concluded that government action to enforce particular provisions of the code is inappropriate. This is because (1) many of the code provisions already have been accepted on a voluntary basis; (2) some of the code's provisions are considered inappropriate in the United States, where social and economic circumstances are different from those in the developing nations which were the primary target of the code; and (3) some provisions of the code are counter to certain US legal and constitutional provisions."

Determining the practical effects of the code is somewhat problematic. Published studies do not address the debated question of whether marketing practices affect decisions concerning feeding mode. Rather, they attempt to evaluate how education about and encouragement of breast-feeding affect the decision to breast-feed or not[8,24,25]. Marketing practices in LDCs have reportedly changed sufficiently that coalition boycotts against formula companies have been discontinued. The role of the WHO code in this cannot be determined; however, the credit appears to belong more to the "grassroots" movements that helped to alert WHO to the breast-feeding issues rather than to the WHO code itself.

Of final note is the effect of the code within the WHO community. The WHO has continued to promote the code, adopted as a recommendation. At the Thirty-Fifth World Health Assembly, it was noted that few member states had adopted and adhered to the international code as a minimum requirement or implemented the code in its entirety. WHO therefore resolved to design and coordinate a program with the aim of supporting member states in their efforts to implement and monitor the code.[20]

SUMMARY

In this chapter we have attempted to explore the content of controversies within the United States preceding and surrounding the WHO International Code of Marketing of Breast-Milk Substitutes. We have attempted to present an objective perspective on these issues and purposefully have avoided making ethical judgments concerning the intent or nature of decisions made at that time. It is our hope that by outlining the issues in this fashion, we have encouraged readers to evaluate these events themselves with a fresh and unbiased approach and to reach their own conclusions with the invaluable assistance of hindsight and historical perspective.

REFERENCES

1. Bain K: The incidence of breastfeeding in hospitals in the United States. *Pediatrics* 1948;2:313–320.
2. Meyer HF: Breastfeeding in the United States: Extent and possible trend. Survey of 1,904 hospitals with two and a quarter million births in 1956. *Pediatrics* 1958;22:116–121.
3. Jellife DV: Social change and infant feeding. *Am J Clin Nutr* 1967;20:279.
4. Jellife DV, Jellife EFP: The urban avalanche and child nutrition II: Special problems in developing countries. *J Am Diet Assoc* 1970;57:114.
5. Jellife DV: Breast milk and the world protein gap. *Clin Pediatr* 1968;7:96.
6. Jellife DV: Commerciogenic malnutrition? *Nutr Rev* 1972;30: 205.
7. World Health Organization: *International Code of Marketing of Breast Milk Substitutes.* Geneva, World Health Organization, 1981.
8. DHHS Task Force: Report of the task force on the scientific evidence relating to infant feeding practices and infant health. *Pediatrics* 1984;74:2.
9. Abrams E: Infant formula code: Why the US may stand alone? *Washington Post,* 1981.
10. *Marketing and Promotion of Infant Formula in Developing Nations,* hearing before the Subcommittee on Health and Scientific Research of the Committee on Human Resources. United States Senate, US Government Printing Office, Washington, DC, 1978.
11. Anderson J: Formula flap: Story behind the lone "no." *Washington Post,* 1981.
12. Board of Directors of the Ambulatory Pediatric Association: The World Health Organization code of marketing of breast-milk substitutes. *Pediatrics* 1981;68:432–434.
13. Lucey JF: Editor's note. *Pediatrics* 1981;68:431.
14. May CD: The infant formula controversy: A notorious threat to reason in matters of health. *Pediatrics* 1981;68:428–430.
15. Ervin SJ Jr: *The Washington Star,* 1981.
16. Mann J: *The Washington Post,* 1981.

17. Lucey JF: Does a vote of 118 to 1 mean the USA was wrong? *Pediatrics* 1981;68:430–431.
18. The Work of World Health Organization, 1973—Annual Report of the Director-General to the World Health Assembly and to the United Nations. Official Records of the World Health Organization No 213, Geneva, 1974, pp 110–111.
19. Twenty-Seventh World Health Assembly: Geneva, May 7–23, 1974. Part II Verbatim Records of Plenary Meetings, Summary Records and Reports of Committees, official records No 218, Geneva, 1974, pp 354–356.
20. Handbook of resolutions and decisions of the World Health Assembly and the Executive Board, Volume II — 26th to 35th World Health Assemblies, 51st to 70th Sessions of the Executive Board, Geneva, 1983, pp 76–79, 204.
21. Thirty-Third World Health Assembly, Geneva, May 5–23, 1980, Summary Records of Committee. Geneva, 1983.
22. Executive Board, Sixty-Seventh Session, Summary Records, Geneva, January 14–30, 1981, p 316.
23. Thirty-Fourth World Health Assembly, Geneva, May 4–22, 1981; Summary Records of Committees, Geneva, 1981, pp 199–200.
24. Jason JM, Nieburg P, Mark JS: Mortality and infectious disease associated with infant-feeding practices in developing countries. *Pediatrics* 1984;74(2):702–727.
25. Narayanan I, Prakash K, Prabhakar AK, et al: A planned prospective evaluation of the anti-infective property of varying quantities of expressed human milk. *Acta Paediatr Scand* 1982;71: 441–445.
26. Butz WP, Habicht JP, DaVanzo J: Environmental factors in the relationship between breast feeding and infant mortality: The role of sanitation and water in Malaysia. *Am J Epidemiol* 1984;119:516–523.
27. Clavano NR: Mode of feeding and its effect on infant mortality and morbidity. *J Trop Pediatr* 1982;28:287–293.
28. Kanaaneh H: The relationship of bottle feeding to malnutrition and gastroenteritis in a pre-industrial setting. *J Trop Pediatr Environ Child Health* 1972;18:302–306.
29. Glass RI, Svennerholm A, Stoll BJ, et al: Milk antibodies protect breast-fed children against cholera. *N Engl J Med* 1983;30: 1389–1392.
30. Infant and young child feeding and international code of marketing of breast milk substitutes. USA Report to the World Health Organization, August 1983. Office of International

Health, Office of the Assistant Secretary of Health, Department of Health and Human Services.

31. Schmidt BJ: Breastfeeding in Sorocaba S. Pauelo, Brazil. Study performed on mothers belonging to different socio-economic levels. *Courrier* 1980;30:561–567.
32. Ekwo EE, Dusdieker LB, Booth BM: Factors influencing initiation of breast-feeding. *Am J Dis Child* 1983;137:375–377.

CHAPTER 10

GROWTH AND DEVELOPMENT OF GIRLS

Isabelle Valadian, MD

INTRODUCTION

Longitudinal studies of growth and development started in the US in the early 1930s. As their participants aged, a life-span perspective emerged. Childhood illness, nutrition and growth became identified as antecedents to, or even determinants of, adult obesity, cardiovascular disease, gynecological health, and reproductive capacity.

In an epidemiological approach to obstetrics, prevention of complications should start in childhood. Unless we improve the health and nutrition of young girls long before menarche, we will not achieve the desired goals of reducing the incidence of low birth weight or infant mortality. This chapter will review the impact of child growth and development on adult health.

Growth is the increase of the dimensions of the body as a whole or its various segments, organs, and tissues. It refers, here, only to increases in size compatible with health, which in sequential changes lead to final adult size. For example, tumors will not be considered as growth. The underlying processes are cell enlargement and multiplication as well as an increase in the intercellular substances. Growth can be measured and expressed in centimeters or inches and pounds or grams in relation to time (defined as age of attainment of certain size).

Development is the sequential change, in function, resulting from maturation processes such as cell differentiation, bone calcification, fusion of the epiphyses with diaphyses and the body's accomodation or adjustment to its environment. Examples are immunologic activities, progress of gross and fine motor coordination appearance, and activities of the secondary sex characteristics. Development is measured by indirect methods and is expressed in scales of defined attainment.

Growth and development are interrelated; at times there may be more growth than development, at other times the reverse. Most of the time it is quite difficult to make a distinction and both are used in tandem.

GROWTH IN HEIGHT AND WEIGHT

Growth is continuous to final adult size. It is continuous but is not constant in amount or uniform in rate of progress. The pattern of human growth has two cycles of rapid growth. Rapid growth is more vulnerable to environmental circumstances and requires, at these periods, closer supervision and a different schedule of examinations. This fact is well appreciated in infant care: traditionally infants are seen monthly in the first year and less frequently in the second year, but this fact is overlooked in the care of the adolescent, although vulnerability has been established. For example, lack of growth in Japanese children happened at every age level during World War II, but the greatest effect was seen in boys 14 years old and girls 12 years old. Since 1948, a steady and rapid increase in height has been seen to occur in these same groups, emphasizing the sensitivity of the adolescent age period.[1]

FIRST CYCLE OF GROWTH

The first cycle of growth covers the prenatal to infancy period. It starts at conception; its accelerating phase is completed before birth, and a decelerating phase extends throughout much of infancy, although this decelerating phase is still the most rapid extrauterine growth.

By the end of the first trimester, the microscopic ovum has grown into a fetus about 10 cm in length and weighing about 15 g; this sounds like small growth quantitatively, but represents a 10,000-fold acquisition of new material. Increase in size in the first trimester is due to creation of tissues (nerve, bone, connective, and muscle) through rapid cell multiplication and differentiation into an organism with most of the gross human anatomic features at 12 weeks. This makes the fetus very vulnerable to intrauterine environmental factors at this time. Physical factors which interfere with oxygenation of the fetus, infections such as toxoplasmosis, cytomegalic inclusion disease, German measles, and other viral and bacterial conditions, and injuries by radiation, trauma, and chemicals, such as quinine and thalidomide, may retard or arrest the development of a given organ resulting in malformation or death. The result depends on the timing of the insult and the nature of the agent.

Emphasis on the importance of this first trimester is essential since at the time when vital organs are being formed, women are often unaware of their pregnancies and, therefore, are not seeking care. Great responsibility rests in the education of prospective mothers in avoiding environmental conditions which are known to damage the embryo.

Growth in length and weight accelerates further after the first trimester; length increments are larger during the second trimester, reaching a peak toward the fifth month, while weight increase predominates during the third trimester, reaching a peak of gain just before term. Premature infants, therefore, may not differ greatly in length, since by the sixth month 80% of mature birth length is attained, but will vary greatly in weight. For this reason birth weight is a better index of prematurity than length at birth, and the term "low-birth-weight infant" is commonly used to describe the premature infant.

The birth of the full-term infant occurs on the decelerating slope of the first cycle of growth. The average length is approximately 50 cm and weight is about 3400 g. From then on, although still growing at a rapid pace, the increments in length and weight per unit of time will diminish. By the end of the first year, the birth length has increased by 50% and the birth weight has tripled.

In the first few days after birth, newborns may actually lose up to 10% of their birth weight, which reflects in large part a reduction of the body's water content. The greatest loss occurs in the first 24 hr, the lowest weight being reached on the third or fourth day; normally the birth weight is regained by the tenth day. There is no indication to increase the fluid intake unless weight loss exceeds 10% or the birth weight is not regained by the fourteenth day.

From the tenth day the rate of weight gain is virtually constant in the first year. Any arrest that persists for two weeks or actual loss signals pathology or deficient feeding. In the first year, weight is a very good indicator of progress, although it should not be taken as the only criterion of health. Gain in weight is greater in the first than in any subsequent year; it increases at a progressively slower rate and with less regularity in subsequent years. It, therefore, provides a much less accurate index of satisfactory progress.

In the preschool years, the decline in weight gain is much greater than that in height gain, resulting in the child appearing thinner; misinterpretation of this normal process often creates anxiety among parents. From the fourth year until adolescence the situation is reversed, the increments in height declining while the rate of weight gain slowly rises; this results in children looking stockier. Overall, this is a period or relatively uniform and slow growth over the entire middle period of childhood.

SECOND CYCLE OF GROWTH

Rapid increments in height and weight occur again at adolescence; this second cycle of growth is known as the adolescent growth spurt. Changes in weight start earlier than changes in height, but gains are less striking and fluctuate more. Changes in height are easier to follow and are more abrupt. A girl who is gaining 2–3 cm per year starts to gain 5–6 cm for a couple of years. After this, she will return to a gain of 5–6 cm and less until her growth stops.

In the second cycle, the accelerating phase starts in the prepubescent stages, reaches a peak where many of the secondary sex characteristics and major physiologic changes occur, and tapers off to cessation of growth at maturity.

ASSESSMENT OF GROWTH

Distribution of a variety of physical measurements obtained from large groups of children are expressed in percentile values or in means and standard deviations. These standards are difficult to use routinely in table form. Given a series of numerical values of an individual child, it is difficult to determine mentally how they differ from the standards. Standards are best used when translated into charts on which lines indicate the sequential changes of the distribution of numerical values with time (mostly chronologic age) for either means and standard deviation or for the 3rd, 10th, 25th, 50th, 75th, 90th and 97th percentiles. Percentile charts developed at the Harvard School of Public Health are based on "distance," that is, on measurement attained at one time by cumulative progress during the preceding years. Other charts are based on velocity, ie, on increments gained from the previous measurement.

The first step in appraising the growth of a child is by comparison with others of the same sex, age, and preferably, of the same ethnic group. There is no specific point in a standard at which normality ends and abnormality begins, but a child at the extremes of the range or outside the range needs further evaluation. A single value of either height or weight tells little about a child's growth. For example, three children of the same age happen to be at the 25th percentile for their weight. One child was always following that percentile line, the second decreased from the 75th percentile, while the third increased up from the 10th percentile. Obviously, the situations are quite different.

Sequential values are necessary to ascertain how a child maintains his relative position from one year to the next; this is the only way to recognize and understand the pattern of growth of an individual child. The importance of sequential values over the years preceding adolescence is further enhanced in adoloescence because it provides a reliable method for locating the upward departure from an established channel of growth and, therefore, it provides a simple way of recognizing the onset of forthcoming changes.

Measurements of a single dimension are of very limited value. For example, a girl at the 25th percentile level for weight cannot be considered undernourished if her height is at the 3rd, 10th, or 25th percentile, but she might be undernourished if her height were at the 75th or 90th. Dimensions, therefore, should be compared; here again, there are no established rules for estimating the difference in position of height and weight, but usually a difference of more than two percentile lines signals further investigation.

BODY GROWTH PATTERN CHARACTERISTIC OF GIRLS

Within the general pattern of growth in height and weight discussed above, girls display distinct common characteristics. These differences begin late in the prenatal period. They are negligible to the 30th week, become more clearly identifiable by the 35th, and gradually increase until full term. Female fetuses grow consistently slower than males in length and weight. Most investigators report differences of about 1–3% in birthlength and 4% in birthweight at term. Sex differences in size at birth are mainly caused by the differences in rate of fetal growth since there are no substantial differences in the duration of gestation between the sexes. They are probably set by the genetic constitution and become manifest when fetal sex hormones begin to have an effect on growth, testosterone having a markedly growth-stimulating effect.

The slower growth of girls continues during the first year of life reaching, on the average, a 500-g difference by one year; thereafter, differences are more modest. Throughout middle childhood, where growth is slow, sex differences are very slight, but they become quite striking in magnitude, speed, and timing during the second cycle of growth. Girls start the second cycle of growth about 1½–2 years earlier than boys; they begin to grow quickly by 10–12 years when most boys still grow slowly and, for a couple of years, girls are taller and heavier: this is only temporary. Later, girls begin to slow down, and boys begin to grow quickly, with a greater growth velocity. This, added to the fact that they had two years more to grow, makes them, on the average, taller than females at maturity.

In general, the physical development of the girls fluctuates less, and they are more resistant to environmental factors. For example, among malnourished children, girls' growth slows down less than boys' and recovers more quickly. War deprivation effects in Guam were apparent in both sexes but less in girls, and children who survived the atomic bomb showed stunting of growth but again, girls less than boys.[2,3] Besides being less vulnerable to environmental insults, girls are also less responsive to favorable changes; for example when socioeconomic conditions improve, height gains are greater, on average, for boys. The physiologic reason of the greater stability of growth among girls is not fully known.

GROWTH OF OTHER BODY COMPONENTS

The pattern for growth in body height and weight is also characteristic of growth of certain tissues, such as bone and muscle, or certain organs, such as those of digestion, respiration, circulation, and excretion. Other tissues and organs follow different growth patterns.

Neural Growth

The central nervous system, the eyes, and much of the auditory system grow rapidly in the fetal period and infancy, more gradually during the middle and later part of the first decade, and decline at a steady rate until sometime after puberty when growth ceases except for a slight increase during the adolescent growth cycle.

Whereas the weight of an infant at birth is only about 5% that of an adult, his brain at birth, weighing approximately 350 g is 25% the weight of the adult brain. The peak rate in the weight gain of the brain takes place just before birth and continues, somewhat less rapidly for the first six months postnatally. About 50% of postnatal growth takes place in the first year of life when the weight is increased by 1000 g, bringing the total size to 70% of the adult size. This timing is well documented by: (1) differences in the number of cells in the brain of normal children who died of accidents and of fetuses removed by therapeutic abortion[4] and multiplication of neuron ends by the time of birth in the cerebral cortex;[5] (2) rapid progress in myelinization around birth,[4] following an orderly sequence through fetal and postnatal life continuing throughout childhood;[6] and (3) increased enzyme activity in the fetal brain related to cytologic changes.[7]

Other studies have demonstrated the vulnerability of the brain to severe malnutrition occurring during that period; malnutrition reduces brain weight and markedly reduces the number of cells.[8] There is evidence that interruption of cell division and myelinization occuring before the 6th month of life may result in permanent deficits within the brain.[8]

Several questions remain to be satisfactorily answered with regard to whether retarded brain growth results in irreversible damage. Some support it, since 90% of growth is achieved before birth and very little is still to be acquired; others challenge this concept.[9] Another important question is whether small size means poor function and mental retardation. This question is the subject of many good studies. Differentiating between malnutrition alone as a cause of deficient mental function and other environmental factors, with or without malnutrition, is difficult. Controversies on this question are summarized in at least three reviews.[10–12] The most significant fact to emerge from these studies is the tremendous importance of prenatal and postnatal nutrition and the primary place nutrition should take in our maternity and infant care services.

Genital Growth

There is little increase of genital growth during early life. The uterus of the fetus grows under the influence of maternal hormones. Their effect decreases after birth and then disappears, so that by six months after birth the uterus is 20% smaller than at birth; the cervix decreases in size more than the corpus. Also at birth there is proliferation of the endometrium and some degree of secretory activities; these disappear after birth.[13] The uterus and ovaries develop rapidly just before and during puberty.[14] Before menarche the cervix grows considerably, looking long in relation to the corpus, its canal becomes larger, and its glands become active. The secretion of the cervical epithelium is mucoid and acquires the characteristics of estrogen stimulation such as formation of fernlike crystals in thin preparation typical of mid-portion ovarian cycle in older girls and adult women.[15] Closer to menarche, the corpus grows in response to estrogen, and soon its length may equal that of the cervix.[15] In the early phase this growth is due primarily to the growth of myometrium and the endometrium,[15] so that the increase in size of the uterus involves both the endometrium and myometrium before menarche.[14]

The vagina increases in length in the premenarche years and its epithelium undergoes cytological changes which usually are the first indication of the forthcoming events of puberty. Preceding menarche, the ovaries grow much faster, the number of large follicles in the various stages of development increases, and probably the oocytes which mature are those already present at birth.[15] The rapid growth of the uterus and ovaries is also vulnerable to environmental factors. Good nutrition in the years before menarche may play an important part in establishing the capacity of a girl to reproduce satisfactorily in later life.[17] The sequence of breast development and other secondary sex characteristics are discussed later.

Lymphoid Growth

The thymus, lymph nodes, tonsils, and follicles of the spleen and lymph tissue of the intestines grow rapidly in childhood resulting, by 8–10 years, in a total mass nearly twice that found in adults. Their growth rate decreases and ceases about the time of puberty. Enlarged tonsils and adenoids of the young child are characteristic of this growth pattern, and will actually shrink.

Adipose Growth

Body fat is estimated by skinfold measurements at the triceps and subcapular areas or by x-rays of the limbs. Correlation is good with more elaborate techniques of measuring fat by displacement, body radiation counts, or the estimation of lean body mass and subtracting it from the weight. All measurements indicate a pattern as follows: Fat increases steadily and quite rapidly for the first nine months after birth and then again at the time of the adolescent growth spurt.[18] This period of maximum growth in height is a good period to help the obese girl lose her fat since fat is not only growing at its minimum rate but actually may even show a loss. The follow-up of the Longitudinal Studies of Child Health and Development revealed that obese adults had been obese children at some periods, but, of the overweight children, it was only those who remained obese after the growth spurt who were most likely to continue to be obese.[17]

Segmental Growth

Different parts of the body grow at different rates, accomplish their growth at different times, and result in changes in body proportions. From conception to infancy the head grows more rapidly than any other part of the body. The growth of the head parallels that of the brain. Reduction in head circumference in children who are malnourished in the first six months of life may reflect the reduced number of cells in the brain.[19] Head circumference in children who are malnourished in the first six months of life may reflect the reduced number of cells in the brain.[19] Head circumference is a very meaningful measurement in the first three to five years only and should be included in health supervision of young children.

DEVELOPMENT, ADAPTATION, AND MATURATION ADJUSTMENT TO EXTRAUTERINE LIFE

The period after birth is a period of adjustment. Many anatomic and physiologic changes, such as the establishment of the respiratory process, occur in less than a second to assure survival. Other changes take place more slowly, with two to four weeks required for attainment of some physiological adjustments, such as the establishment of adequate circulation. There is considerable variation in the efficiency with which individual babies adapt. The important thing is to know what to expect and to recognize what phenomena are within the limits of variability. Skilled observers are needed to detect trouble at its beginning because the distinction between pathology and the extremes of normal phenomena may be very slight. This is a very hazardous period. The first few hours of life are more hazardous than the first three days, which, in turn, are more hazardous than the rest of the first month.

Neuromuscular Development

Parallel to the rapid increase in size in infancy is a rapid maturation of the central nervous system and an increase in muscular function. Neuromuscular functioning involves the whole body of the young and is an important indicator of development and integrity of neuromuscular control. The newborn moves without coordination or specification of movement and has reflex responses to assure survival. Maturation and the exercise of neuromuscular structures unfold coordinated functional patterns such as the ability to reach with the hand, grasp and manipulate objects, or to raise the head, roll over, sit erect, creep, stand, and walk. Detailed knowledge is established on the age sequences of these changes for average children;[20] more recently, knowledge has been established for slow, average, and rapidly maturing infants.[21] Simplified milestones such as the Denver Developmental Tests are useful for screening purpose. Skills are mastered through repetitive exercises in play or some more formal setting.

Skeletal Development

In the fetus, bones are laid down as cartilage. Through biological and chemical processes, fibrous tissue and cartilage are transformed into bones. Bone tissue is radiopaque, while cartilage is not, so that the earliest stages of the ossification process are clearly visible on x-ray film. The process begins at about the fifth fetal month and continues throughout childhood. Ossification proceeds in a constant order among children of all races, first in the clavicle, then in the skull, the long bones, and the spine. The size, shape, and outline on x-ray film of ossification centers can be described; their changes follow a very orderly sequence of features common to most children at a given age. Age–specific descriptions for the average child are used to describe skeletal development.[22]

The film of an individual child is compared with a standard film matched for age and sex; this determines skeletal age based on deviations in months or years from the expected level for chronologic age. There are standards for different segments of the body, including the knee and the foot, but the standard of the hand and wrist is the most practical because of the multiplicity of ossification centers in the region and the relative safety with which this region can be exposed to x-ray. Skeletal maturation in the prenatal period is more rapid for girls than boys. It accelerates long before puberty and is characteristic of an early growth spurt.

SECONDARY SEX CHARACTERISTICS

Tanner[14] describes five stages of breast and pubic hair development. These form a standard for evaluation of an in-

Table 10-1
Stages of Breast and Pubic Hair Development in Girls

Breasts	Stage	Pubic hair
Prepubescent; evaluation of papilla only	I	Prepubescent, no pubic hair
Breast "bud" stage; enlargement of areolar diameter, evaluation of breast and papilla as a small mound	II	Sparse, pale, fine, straight hair appears, chiefly among the labia
Further enlargement of breast and areola	III	Darker, coarser, more curled; begins to spread over pubic area
Projection of areola and papilla to form a secondary mound above the breast level	IV	Hair is adult in type, but does not cover as great an area
Mature stage; areola recedes to the general breast contour, so only the papilla projects.	V	Adult in quantity, type, and horizontal distribution pattern as an inverse triangle

dividual girl's progress toward maturity and are summarized in Table 10-1. Duration of stages and progression from one stage to the other exceeds the variability in onset. Some pass rapidly through all stages in 18–24 months, others linger, taking up to four to five years to reach adult stages. Reports vary as to the most common sequence,[23,24] although differences in methodology may account for these differences.

Menarche is a mature point in the development of the uterus, but does not indicate the fulfillment of reproductive function. Menstrual cycles following menarche may be quite irregular and vary in the amount of flow and accompanying symptoms. The characteristics of the early menstrual periods relate to the future gynecological health of young women.[25,26] Frequently early menstrual periods are anovulatory; adolescent sterility or partial sterility may be seen in the first year or year and a half after menarche. But here again there is a wide range of individual variation, and ovulatory cycles may account for about 50% of all cycles in the two years after menarche, becoming more or less regular after five years.[27,28]

Timing of Sexual Development in Relation to Physical Growth

The development of breasts and pubic hair occurs rather late in relation to the growth spurt in height. Menarche on the other hand, has a close and more constant relationship. It occurs after the year of maximum growth in the decelerating phase of the growth spurt in height. Tallness or shortness may be considered a problem not only by the adolescent girl, but also by her mother, especially if she herself had been unhappy with her size. One should help the girl not only to accept her final size but to like it, to see its advantages, and to understand that it is a relative rather than an absolute matter. The desirable height of adult women is more a question of fashion in society, a cultural attitude. In summary, it is only through a greater understanding and thereby improvement in the nutrition and health of young girls that we can reduce complications during the reproductive years.

REFERENCES

1. Mitchell HS: Protein limitations and human growth. *J Am Diet Assoc* 1964;4:165.
2. Greulich WW: The growth and developmental status of Guamaian children in 1947. *Am J Physiol Anthropol* 1971;9:55–70.
3. Greulich WW, Crismon CS, Turner ML: The physical growth and development of children who survived the atomic bombing of Hiroshima and Nagasaki. *J Pediatr* 1953;43:121–145.
4. Winnick M: Nucleic acid and protein content during growth of the human brain. *Pediatr Res* 1968;2:352.

5. Conel J: The Postnatal Development of the Human Cerebral Cortex. Cambridge, MA, Harvard Press, 1963, vol I-VII.
6. Aguilar JJ, Williamson M: Observations on the growth and development of the brain, in Cheek DB (ed): *Human Growth: Body Composition, Cell Growth and Intelligence.* Philadelphia, Lea and Febiger, 1968.
7. Cheek DB, Migeon CJ, Millitts EP: The concept of biologic age, in Cheek DB (ed): *Human Growth: Body Composition, Cell Growth and Intelligence.* Philadelphia, Lea and Febiger, 1968.
8. Winnick M, Rosso F: Effects of severe early malnutrition in cellular growth of human brain. *Pediatr Res* 1969;3:181.
9. Cheek DB: Effect of fetal malnutrition on brain is questioned. *Pediatr New* 1971;5.
10. Cravioto J, DiLicardie EF, Birch HG: Nutrition, growth and neurointegrative development: An experimental and ecologic study. *Pediatrics (Suppl)* 1966;38:2.
11. Coursin D: Relationship of nutrition to central nervous system development and function. *Fed Proc* 1957;27:134.
12. Frisch RE: Present status of the supposition that malnutrition causes permanent mental retardation. *Am J Clin Nutr* 1970;53(2): 189.
13. Ober W, Bernstein J: Observations on the endometrium and ovary in the newborn. *Pediatrics* 1955;16:445.
14. Tanner JM: *Growth at Adolescence.* Oxford, England, Blackwell Scientific Publications, 1962.
15. Marshall WA, Tanner JM: Puberty, in Davis JA, Dobbing J (eds): *Scientific Foundation of Pediatrics,* ed 2, 1984, p 177.
16. Valadian I, Reed RB: Influence of nutrition factors during early adolescence on reproductive efficiency, in Janerich DT, Skalko RG, Porter IH (eds): *Congenital Defects, New Directions in Research.* New York, Academic Press, 1974, pp 57–71.
17. Valadian I, Berkey C, Reed RB: *Adolescent Nutrition As It Relates To Cardiovascular Disease and Reproductive Capacity Later in Life.* Marabou Symposium on Nutrition in Adolescence. Sundyberg, Sweden, 1980, pp 75–79.
18. Tanner JM: Radiographic studies of body composition in children and adults, in Brovzek J (ed): *Human Body Composition.* Oxford, England, Pergamon Press, 1965, p 211.
19. Winnick M, Rosso P: Head circumference and cellular growth of the brain in normal and marasmic children. *J Pediatr* 1969;74: 744.
20. Gesell A, et al: *The First Five Years of Life.* New York, Harper, 1940.

21. Brazelton T: *Infants and Mothers.* New York, Delacorte Press, 1970.
22. Greulich WW, Pyle IS: *Radiographic Atlas of Skeletal Development of the Hand and Wrist,* ed 2. Stanford University Press, 1959.
23. Faust MS: Somatic development of adolescent girls. *Monogr Soc Res Child Dev* 1977;42:1–90.
24. Marshall WA, Tanner JM: Variation in the pattern of pubertal changes in girls. *Arch Dis Child* 1969;44:291.
25. Gardner J: Adolescent menstrual characteristics as predictors of gynecological outcome. *Ann Hum Biol* 1983;10(1):31.
26. Gardner J, Valadian I: Changes over thirty years in an index of gynecological health. *Ann Hum Biol* 1983;10(1):41–55.
27. Apter D: Serum steroids and pituitary hormones in female puberty: A partly longitudinal study. *Clin Endocrinol* 1980;12:107.
28. Lemarchand-Berand TH, Zufferey MM, Reymond M, et al: Maturation of the hypothalamo-pituitary-ovarian axis in adolescent girls. *J Clin Endocrinol Metab* 1982;54:241.

CHAPTER 11

INTRODUCTORY STATISTICS FOR OBSTETRICIANS

Timothy Heeren, PhD

INTRODUCTION

With the current emphasis on medical research, an overwhelming number of medical journals present results from scientific studies. These studies follow a variety of experimental designs, each with certain strengths and weaknesses. Results are usually presented in a statistical format using statistical terminology and notation. Further, two or more studies investigating the same question often reach what seem to be conflicting or contradictory conclusions. The task of assimilating the information from these articles can be difficult. The goal of this chapter is to help the clinician evaluate and weigh, from a statistical vantage point, the information presented in medical articles. This chapter will be more concerned with the understanding of experimental and statistical results than with the selection of an appropriate statistical procedure or the "how-to" aspects of performing a statistical test (although Section 8 describes the chi-square test of independence in some detail).

Many questions may be addressed by a scientific article. For example, is a new treatment more effective, is a factor associated with a specific outcome, or what patient characteristics are associated with a particular condition? Studies may follow various designs, that is, there are different ways of assembling a sample and collecting data to address a question. Observational, cross-sectional, case–control, and prospective designs are commonly used in medical research. This chapter will focus on one particular research situation, the comparison of two treatments (or the comparison of a treatment to a placebo) with respect to their effectiveness in preventing an adverse outcome, and the designs relevant to this situation. However, the discussion that follows can be generalized to other experimental situations.

This chapter is not intended to be a complete discussion of the statistical issues involved in comparing two treatments. Rather, it is intended to give a general understanding of (1) the issues of design and sample selection that may affect the reliability of a study, (2) the aspects of a statistical test that may influence the confidence behind a particular result, and (3) an understanding of the chi-square test of independence.

TREATMENT OF PROM, AN EXAMPLE

To illustrate the issues involved in evaluating and interpreting a medical study, we present summaries of three articles dealing with the use of steroids in treating premature rupture of the membrane (PROM) in the preterm pregnancy. All three articles represent good scientific research and present results clearly. Taken chronologically, they also illustrate the development of medical knowledge. And, of course, these studies reach different conclusions.

First some background on the treatment of PROM, from the introductions of the articles to be presented. It is generally accepted that the optimal management of PROM after 34–36 weeks of gestation, when fetal lung maturity can be expected, is immediate delivery. At the time of these studies, there was controversy as to the best course of action when PROM occurs earlier in the pregnancy. In this situation, there were traditionally two strategies to choose between: (1) a policy of watchful waiting, which runs the risk of ascending infection and amnionitis, and (2) induced labor, which runs the risk of prematurity and the development of respiratory distress syndrome (RDS) in the infant after delivery. A third strategy includes the use of corticosteroid therapy in accelerating fetal lung maturity. However, PROM may differ from premature labor with respect to the efficacy and safety of steroids. For instance, steroids may aggravate infection or alter host immune responses in both mother and neonate. The following studies investigated the effectiveness of corticosteroid treatment for patients with PROM compared to the treatment of expectant management. Our discussion will be focused on one outcome, the development of RDS in the infant.

The Vermont study[1], published in 1977, presents data collected between 1974 and 1976 at the Medical Center of Vermont. The abstract follows:

> Of 43 women admitted with premature rupture of the membranes between 27 and 32 weeks' gestation, 27 received antepartum glucocorticoid with delivery timed to occur approximately 24 h after the first dose of steroid. Sixteen patients did not receive glucocorticoid and were managed expectantly. Neonatal mortality was significantly less in the steroid group (15% vs 50%, $P < 0.01$), and this difference was explained by a reduction in deaths from respiratory distress syndrome. Rates of infectious morbidity for both mothers and infants were similar between the steroid-treated group and the group managed expectantly.

Some additional information from the article is useful. The authors describe their study as a retrospective study. The treatment group received 6 mg of betamethasone on admission and again 12 h later. While an attempt was made to deliver patients receiving steroids 24 h after the first dose, in seven cases delivery occurred before 24 h.

The control group was managed with bed rest awaiting the onset of spontaneous labor. Some patients in each treatment group were transferred from other hospitals with membranes that had ruptured more than 24 h earlier. The treatment a patient received was decided on by the attending physician after a discussion with the patient; no information is given on the factors that may have influenced the decision. The incidence of RDS was 22% (6 of 21 patients) in the group treated with steroids, and 81% (13 of 16) in the group managed expectantly. This difference is statistically significant at $P < 0.001$; the evidence suggests that steroid treatment is effective in reducing the risk of RDS in preterm infants with PROM.

The Melbourne study[2] was published in 1979. This study was based on data collected between 1976 and 1978 at the Royal Women's Hospital in Melbourne. The abstract follows:

> In a consecutive series of 93 patients with premature rupture of the membranes at 20 to 34 weeks of gestation, the perinatal mortality was 23.7%. One quarter of the deaths were due to lethal congenital abnormalities. Eighteen percent were due to intrauterine infection, and 36% resulted from severe respiratory distress syndrome (RDS). Corticosteroid therapy increased the risk of infection, especially in patients with cervical incompetence, and did not reduce the incidence or severity of RDS. Almost one third of the patients were delivered within 48 hours of membrane rupture; however, short-term treatment with salbutamol was able to dclay the delivery for at least six days in 5 of the 13 patients to whom it was given. As postponement of delivery for days or weeks after the membranes have ruptured reduces the incidence and severity of RDS, this therapy may well have a place in the treatment of this condition.

This is a prospective study. Patients were alternately assigned to either the treatment or control group, although

40% of the subjects were private patients whose physicians were not bound by the study protocol. However, the authors report that these physicians generally accepted the assignment scheme. The treatment group received 4 mg of betamethasone every 8 hr up to a total of 24 mg, unless delivery occurred before completion of therapy. Delivery may have occurred many weeks after the time of membrane rupture. No attempt was made to induce labor; labor was inhibited when it commenced simultaneously during the 48 hr of steroid administration. The control group was managed under a policy of watchful expectancy. The incidence of RDS for patients from 25 to 34 weeks of gestation was 57% (12 of 21 patients) for the group receiving steroids and 58% (21 of 36 patients) for the control group. This difference is not statistically significant; the conclusion is that steroid treatment has no effect on the incidence of RDS in infants from preterm pregnancies with PROM.

The California Study,[3] published in 1981, presents data collected between 1977 and 1980 at the University of California-Irvine Medical Center and at Women's Hospital, Long Beach. The abstract follows:

> A prospective randomized study involving patients with premature rupture of the membranes between the twenty-eighth week and the thirty-fourth week of pregnancy was conducted. Patients with chorioamnionitis, advanced labor, and fetal distress, as well as those with mature lecithin/sphingomyelin ratios and/or Gram stains positive for bacteria, were delivered immediately. The remaining patients were randomized. One group received betamethasone. Tocolytic agents were used in this group when necessary. After 48 hours all patients given corticosteroids (CS group) were delivered. The second group was managed expectantly (EM group) and were delivered only when spontaneous labor or infection occurred. A total of 160 patients were randomized, 80 in each group. Maternal outcomes, including chorioamnionitis and cesarean section rates, were not different; however the endometritis rate

> was significantly higher in the CS group ($P < 0.05$). Neonatal outcome did not differ in mean birth weights, perinatal death rates, neonatal infections or incidence of respiratory distress. The frequency of prolonged hospital stay (>4 weeks) was higher in the neonates in the CS group ($P < 0.01$). The conclusion is that corticosteroids and active management in patients with premature rupture of the membranes and premature gestations do not decrease the incidence of respiratory distress syndrome or perinatal mortality and may aggravate certain infectious complications.

Patients in the steroid group were given two 12-mg doses of betamethasone 24 hr apart. Tocolysis was used when regular contractions occurred. All patients were delivered at the end of the 48-hr period, either by discontinuing the tocolytic agent, by inducing labor, or by cesarean section. No statistically significant difference was observed in the rates of RDS; observed rates were 17% (14 of 80 patients) in the steroid group and 21% (17 of 79) in the control group.

A clinician, interested in the treatment of PROM in the preterm pregnancy, is presented with the above information. Three studies investigated the same basic question, but reached different conclusions. How should the evidence from each study be weighed when integrating the information from these articles? Given the body of evidence, do we conclude that steroid treatment is effective or ineffective?

EVALUATION OF A STATISTICAL STUDY

Statistical studies may be evaluated on two sets of criteria. The first involves issues of design, that is, how subjects (patients) were selected for study, how they were assigned to a particular treatment, and how data was collected on subjects. The second set of concerns involves issues of analysis, such as how statistical results are reported and how results should be interpreted. Ideally, a study sample should be assembled and data collected with the aim of answering a specific question. While this seems reasonable, there are many studies that do not follow this ideal. Indeed, there are times when it may not be appropriate to meet this ideal. The reliability of a study is dependent on sample selection, randomization of patients, specifics of treatment, and data collection.

The second issue is that of analysis. We will focus on understanding the terminology and notation of statistics, and the underlying framework of a statistical test of hypothesis. When comparing two treatments, finding a statistical difference between treatments is a strong result and carries different weight than finding no statistical difference between treatments.

This chapter will not address such questions as whether the techniques used are appropriate or whether data are presented fairly and accurately. The improper use of statistics is less of a concern today than it once was, thanks to the increasing use of statistics and the attention given to statistical detail in the review process. Nonetheless, inappropriate use of statistical techniques still occurs. Some of the more common errors involve the improper analysis of repeated measurements or dependent samples, the use of techniques when their underlying assumptions are strongly violated, and ignoring problems associated with multiple comparisons. But these issues are the responsibility of reviewers. The reader should be able to trust that the methods are appropriate and that the results are accurately presented.

A third set of issues also needs to be addressed when critiquing a scientific study, but these are not issues for the statistician. The clinician must ask such questions as whether or not the patient population under study is clearly defined and appropriate, whether the details of the treatment protocol are appropriate, and whether care given to the patients other than the treatments of interest may affect outcome. In other words, the quality of the medicine must be evaluated. It is the responsibility of the author to provide enough information for the reader to make this evaluation. The appropriateness of the medical science should be determined before moving on to the issues of design and analysis.

Study Design

In statistics, the term "experimental design" refers to the way data are obtained. How was the sample of subjects chosen? How were subjects assigned to treatments? How were outcomes evaluated? These are issues that relate to the quality of the data collected, rather than the actual interpretation of the data. If the data were not collected in a way that allows fair comparison of treatments, then any conclusion must be held suspect, regardless of its statistical strength. One way to classify a design is by whether or not the subjects were under treatment when the study question was posed. Retrospective studies go back in time, through record review or other means, to gather an historical sample. Prospective studies assemble the sample and collect data while subjects are under study.

A retrospective study is usually the first step in the investigation of a research question. Retrospective studies make use of past experience and data on patients already treated, so there is no delay waiting for a sample of patients to accumulate. The economy, both in terms of time and money, of a retrospective study is one of the major advantages of such studies. However, there are dangers when dealing with retrospective data. In order to fairly compare two treatments, the subjects assigned to each treatment must be similar, otherwise differences observed between treatment groups might be due to differences between the patients rather than differences between the treatments. In most retrospective studies, the question of interest was not posed when the patients were treated, and patients were assigned to treatment without any thought of comparing treatments. When a physician assigns one patient to one treatment and another patient to some other treatment, there is usually a reason. These patients may differ on factors that could affect treatment outcome. This is referred to as selection bias. Differences observed between treatment groups may be attributable to the bias in selecting patient groups rather than differences between treatments.

A second concern with retrospective studies also stems from the fact that treatment was not assigned for the purpose of study. The specifics of treatment, such as dose of some drug, time schedule of treatment, or additional medication and care may vary from patient to patient. Ideally, a well-defined protocol should be studied. When treatment is not under study, there is little reason for a strict protocol to be shared by a group of physicians or even followed from patient to patient by the same physician.

Because of these concerns, investigators should provide a description of each treatment sample when presenting a retrospective study. To evaluate the strength of a study, the reader needs to know how similar or how different the treatment groups were. But caution is warranted regardless. Even if groups seem comparable on factors of importance, there may be some subtle selection bias in effect. As a result, retrospective studies are often viewed as preliminary, and investigators often warn of the limitations of this study design when presenting their findings.

A second type of study design used when comparing two treatments is the prospective design with the randomized, blinded clinical trial as the ideal. In a prospective study, a set of questions is formulated and a sample of patients is assembled while the study is underway. Patients are assigned to treatment with the intention of comparing treatments, and so steps may be taken to ensure comparability between treatment groups. Protocols may be established at the start of the study to ensure consistency of treatment. Care may be taken to minimize the risk of bias in evaluating patient outcome.

A prospective study offers the opportunity to minimize the risk of selection bias and possible confounding due to treatment variation; however, not all prospective studies take full advantage of this opportunity. Several points should be considered when evaluating a prospective study. First, does the study have well-defined inclusion and exclusion criteria specifying the population under study? Often treatment will have little effect on patients with very high or very low risk of outcome, and so these patients may not be included in the study. Also, there may be some patients for whom one treatment is more appropriate than the other, and exclusion criteria will ensure these patients receive proper care. Second, does the study have a formal rule for assignment of patients to treatment? The ideal here is some form of randomized assignment following subject consent. The purpose of an assignment scheme is to minimize selection bias. Patient consent is required to avoid problems of patient refusal. For instance, suppose some patients who are assigned treatment A refuse this treatment and so receive B. This may introduce a bias. Including these patients includes a type of patient under B that is not included under A, while excluding these patients excludes a type of patient from A who is not excluded from B. Third, a well-defined treatment protocol should be stated to minimize variation in outcome due to variation in treatment. Fourth, where appropriate, subjects and investigators should be kept blind, that is, the treatment a subject receives should not be known by the subject or the investigator evaluating the subject. This is to minimize the possibility of bias in auxiliary care or in the evaluation of outcome.

Another type of study is the exploratory study. While this design is rarely used in the comparison of two treatments, secondary analyses performed in such studies are often exploratory. Data are explored to see if some factor, such as an auxiliary treatment or patient characteristic, is associated with outcome or perhaps with the effectiveness of one of the treatments under study. Specific hypotheses focused on specific variables have not been formed, rather the data are allowed to suggest as well as test hypotheses.

There are two dangers to an exploratory design. The first is that, like a retrospective study, the sample was not collected with the aim of studying the factors or auxiliary treatments that are being examined. Selection bias may be responsible for observed differences. A second danger to an exploratory design is the more subtle issue of multiple comparisons. Statistical procedures are based on flagging unlikely differences between groups. What is an unlikely difference when making one comparison may not be so unlikely a difference when making many comparisons. (A logical parallel is that, if a person is randomly selected, it is unlikely that he or she will be taller than 6′2″. However, if a sample of 20 people is randomly selected, it is not unlikely that the tallest person in the sample will be at least 6′2″.) As a result, conclusions from exploratory studies must be viewed critically. These studies are often thought of as hypothesis-generating in that they suggest associations rather than formally test a hypothesis.

The above comments can now be put into a practical perspective. A well-designed prospective study is more sound, scientifically, than an exploratory or retrospective study. This is not to say exploratory and retrospective studies should not be done or that the results of these studies should be dismissed. Exploratory studies are often the first step in investigating factors associated with some outcome; to mount a multiyear trial to prospectively collect data before retrospectively examining historical data would be foolish. But the reader, when weighing the results of a particular study, should be aware of the potential strengths and weaknesses of the design and should be able to judge how well the investigators met these issues.

Design of Studies on Treatment of PROM

To illustrate the issues of experimental design, consider the three studies on the use of steroid treatment in the management of PROM. The first point to note is that there are substantial differences in the specifics of steroid treatment across the studies. The dose and timing of steroids differs considerably. While the Vermont and California studies pair steroid treatment with timed delivery at 24 and 48 hr, respectively, the Melbourne study made no attempt to induce labor in patients treated with steroids. The implication of treatment differences must be considered.

The Vermont study was one of the first to focus on the use of steroids in this situation, and so appropriately followed a retrospective design. The authors, in describing the study as a "preliminary report," acknowledge the limitations of this design. Treatment was well defined and consistent within treatment groups. Patients were assigned to treatment "by the responsible attending physician after a frank discussion with the patient." Treatment was not assigned for the purpose of evaluating treatment, and there is no evidence of any effort being made to guarantee patient comparability between treatments. While the patient population is well defined (all patients presenting), patients may be very different with respect to risk of RDS. A related point is that no exclusion criteria are presented. Often a patient is not truly eligible for both treatments, and so should be excluded from study. For example, a woman presenting in advanced labor may not have been eligible for steroid treatment, and so including such patients in the control group may bias the sample.

Some description of the two treatment samples is presented, showing that the samples are similar with respect to birth weight and gestational age, but differ in the proportion of women with PROM more than 24 hr prior to delivery. This suggests possible selection bias against the expectant management group. The benefits of expectant management are in delaying delivery. Yet only 31% of those patients managed expectantly delivered more than 24 hr after PROM, compared to 74% of the steroid patients. No description of age or parity was given.

Overall, this is a well-presented retrospective study. The reader is given enough information to be aware of the limitations of the data. While differences were observed between treatment groups, it may be that these differences were due to differences between patients receiving each treatment rather than the treatments themselves. This study presents support for, rather than proof of, the effectiveness of steroid treatment in preterm PROM.

The Melbourne and California studies both follow a prospective sampling design, with patients allocated to treatment for the purpose of comparing treatments. However, the studies differ on several points of design. The Melbourne study makes use of an informally enforced, arbitrary assignment scheme, while the California study follows a formal randomization scheme where patients are first screened for consent and then randomized to treatment. While the alternating patient assignment scheme is quite reasonable in theory, in practice it may have several drawbacks. A major criticism is that an investigator knows before a patient enters the study which treatment will be assigned. This knowledge may affect his decision whether or not to include the patient in the study. (One benefit of proper exclusion criteria is that they eliminate cases where there may be any hesitation to follow protocol.) Another drawback with any informal scheme is that those less involved in the study may find it easy to break protocol. The more formal the assignment scheme, the less the chance of some unintentional bias sneaking into the study. A related point is that the Melbourne study makes no mention of patients who refused the assigned treatment. Perhaps this never occurred, but it is possible that a woman whose assignment would have been to the steroid group requested the standard treatment. To include this woman in the control group introduces selection bias; to exclude her from the study also introduces selection bias in that had she been assigned to the control group initially, she would not have refused treatment.

Both studies present inclusion and exclusion criteria. Both studies excluded patients in advanced labor at the time of membrane rupture. In addition, the California study excluded patients with chorioamnionitis or fetal distress, as well as patients where the fetus showed evidence of lung maturity. The purpose of exclusion criteria is to identify patients who are not equally eligible for both treatments and ensure these patients receive proper care. Proper exclusion criteria can also minimize problems an investigator may have in arbitrarily assigning patients. It is of interest to note that while the two studies reach similar conclusions, the overall level of RDS is quite different between the two studies: 58% in the Melbourne study compared to 19% in the California study. This may be due to differences in the patient populations, but may in part be due to the stricter exclusion criteria eliminating high-risk patients from the California study.

Given the nature of the treatments, neither the patient or the attending physician can be blind to treatment. However, in the California study, the radiologist evaluating RDS was blinded, minimizing any possible bias in evaluating outcome.

Even though both studies assigned patients in a way that should minimize differences between treatment groups, it is possible that, by chance, the groups differ on some important factor. Description of the groups should be given. The California study compared groups as to gestational age, maternal age, parity, duration of PROM, and uterine activity. The Melbourne paper offered no such comparison (although, in fairness, the paper was not so focused on the use of steroids).

In summary, the Vermont study followed a retrospective design. Results from this study should be viewed cautiously, since treatment differences may be confounded by patient differences. Both the California and Melbourne studies follow a strong, prospective design. However, the California study was more formally administered and somewhat better documented, at least in the comparison of treatments.

One final note in reference to secondary analysis. While both the Melbourne and California studies were designed to prospectively investigate the effectiveness of steroid treatment on mortality and RDS, both articles address other issues as well. For example, the Melbourne abstract reports that treatment with salbutamol delayed delivery in five of 13 patients and that patients with cervical incompetence may be at higher risk of infection when given corticosteroids. The California abstract reports that endometritis was significantly higher in the steroid group. These statements represent secondary, exploratory analyses, and are subject to concerns of multiple comparisons and, for the salbutamol results, concerns of selection bias. These secondary results must therefore be viewed more critically.

Statistical Analysis

Design issues are fundamental, since they relate to the quality of the data collected. As we just saw, it is important to design a study in a way that allows meaningful comparison of treatments, in order to properly interpret the data. Statistics is the branch of mathematics concerned with making statements about a population based on information from a sample. The Melbourne study, for example, is based on a sample of 93 particular patients, but the conclusions are meant to extend to the treatment of patients in general. There is always some uncertainty in extrapolating from a sample to a larger population, and the field of statistics is concerned with accounting for this uncertainty.

One important factor when interpreting sample results is sample size. A larger sample contains more information about a population, and so provides greater confidence in the sample results and greater precision when generalizing to the population. Statistical tests may be thought of as weighing the strength of a sample result by the same size to determine whether there is sufficient confidence that the result holds for the entire population.

A test of hypotheses is the formal statistical procedure for choosing between two possible conclusions about a population, based on information from a sample. When comparing two treatments with respect to some adverse outcome either (1) the treatments do not differ with respect to their effect on the outcome or (2) one treatment is more effective than the other in reducing the likelihood of the outcome. In statistical terminology statement (1) is the null hypothesis. Generally, the null hypothesis is a statement of no difference between groups or no association between factors. Statement (2) is referred to as the alternative, or research, hypothesis.

The logic underlying a statistical test of hypothesis is to compare the observed sample with what would be expected if the null hypothesis were true. If the observed sample strongly contradicts the null hypothesis, we conclude that the null hypothesis is probably false and therefore the alternative is true. If the observed sample does not strongly contradict the null hypothesis (which does not necessarily mean the sample supports the null), then the null is accepted. As a consequence of this logic, the statistical conclusion that two treatment groups differ is a strong statement and is referred to as a significant result. The statistical conclusion of no treatment difference does not necessarily imply strong evidence of no treatment difference and is therefore called a weak, or nonsignificant, result. When a nonsignificant conclusion is reached, additional information is needed to evaluate how strongly the null hypothesis is supported.

Restated, there are three sample situations that may arise, but only two conclusions that can be reached. Either (1) the sample strongly suggests the null is false, (2) the sample strongly suggests the null is true, or (3) the sample is inconclusive, perhaps due to small sample size, and does not strongly support either hypothesis. Statistical tests reject the null only when (1) occurs. If either (2) or (3) occurs, the null hypothesis is accepted. Therefore, just knowing that there is no statistical difference between treatments does not specify whether the sample is inconclusive or whether the sample strongly supports the hypothesis of no difference.

Formally, a statistical test is concerned with the agreement between a sample and the null hypothesis. This agreement is measured through the probability, or likelihood, of observing such a sample if the null were true. This probability is referred to as the *P-value.* A low *P* value, conventionally *P* less than 0.05 ($P < 0.05$) indicates the sample strongly disagrees with the null, and so the null hypothesis is rejected. When comparing two treatment groups, a *P* value less than 0.05 means that, if there were, in fact, no difference between groups, the chance of observing the sample differences is less than 5 in 100. The hypothesis of no difference is doubted, and so one concludes that there is a difference between groups. A large *P* value indicates that the difference observed in the sample could be due to chance alone, and so the null hypothesis is accepted.

The smaller the *P* value, the stronger the evidence against the null hypothesis. By convention, results tend to be reported at certain "levels of significance." "$P < 0.001$" is a stronger statement than "$P < 0.01$," which is a stronger statement than "$P < 0.05$." Occasionally, studies will report results as significant, or perhaps suggestive, when the *P* value is less than 0.10. Nonsignificant results are often represented as "$P > 0.05$" or "NS."

Statistical Results of Studies on PROM

To illustrate the interpretation of statistical results, we again look at the studies on the use of steroids in the treatment of PROM. The Vermont study showed a significant difference in the incidence of RDS between the two treatment groups, which was 22% in the steroid group and 81% in the expectant management group. Significance was reported as

$P < 0.001$, which implies that, if in fact there was no difference in the underlying risk of RDS for the two groups, the chance of observing such an extreme difference in a sample is less than 1 in 1000. Even though the study is based on only 43 patients, it offers strong evidence that the groups differ (although the design allows questions as to whether or not this difference is due to treatment).

Both the Melbourne and California studies found no significant difference between treatments. These are weak statements, which do not by themselves present convincing evidence of no treatment differences. Some further description incorporating sample size considerations is necessary to allow the reader to weigh the strength of these results. While both studies found remarkably similar rates of RDS under the two treatments, the samples are small enough (21 given steroids in the Melbourne study) so that the results may not be conclusive.

Chi-Square Test of Independence

The statistical procedure used in each of the studies on PROM will be described in this section. To determine an appropriate statistical analysis, an experimental situation can be classified according to the hypotheses being posed and the type of data being used to investigate the hypotheses. Two of the more common general hypotheses are whether or not a difference exists between two or more groups, or whether there is a relationship between two or more factors or outcomes. Data may be classified as a measurement, ordinal, or categorical scale. (For example, to compare two groups on measurement data, the *t* test may be appropriate. To investigate the association between two ordinal scales, Spearman's rank correlation may be used.)

We are interested in comparing two groups on a dichotomous variable. A dichotomous variable is a categorical variable with only two possible outcomes, in this case whether or not an infant develops RDS. The chi-square (χ^2) test of independence is appropriate when comparing groups on a categorical factor. The null hypothesis is that no difference exists between groups with respect to the factor, while the alternative hypothesis is that the groups somehow differ. The chi-square is often called a nondirectional test because the alternative hypothesis does not specify how the groups differ or which treatment is superior.

The chi-square test is applicable in other situations where questions focus on categorical data as well and is one of the most commonly used statistical procedures. However, the test is only appropriate when certain conditions, the assumptions of the test, are met. One condition is that the sample taken was random and that treatment subsamples are independent. There should be no pairing of observations between or within treatment groups. Each subject can appear in the sample only once. If a subject is given treatment A, say, then that subject has not been given treatment B, and is not repeated again under treatment A. Studies where the observations can be paired in other ways, such as a sibling study where one sib receives treatment A, the other B, also violate this assumption. (McNemar's paired sample test of proportions may be appropriate in such situations.)

A second condition necessary for the chi-square test to be reliable is that the samples must be reasonably large. When applied to small samples, the chi-square test tends to exaggerate significance. As a check on sample size, it is often required that expected frequencies (defined below) should be at least five. (When samples are too small for the chi-square test to be reliable, either the chi-square test with Yates' correction or Fisher's exact test may be appropriate.)

The null hypothesis of the chi-square test is that there is no difference between treatments with respect to the proportion developing the outcome. The test is based on a chi-square statistic that measures the difference between the observed sample and what would be expected if, in fact, the

Table 11-1
Two-Way (Contingency) Table

	RDS	No RDS	Total
Steroid group	6 (22%)	21	27
Control group	13 (81%)	3	16
Total	19 (44%)	24	43

null hypothesis were true. The test procedure is illustrated using data from the Vermont study. Table 11-1, referred to as a "two-way" or "contingency" table, categorizes patients according to treatment group and RDS status.

Of 27 patients in the steroid group, 6 developed RDS. Of 16 patients in the control group, 13 developed RDS. Overall, 19 of 43, or 44% of the patients developed RDS. If there is no underlying difference between the steroid and control groups, and ignoring sampling variation, we would expect 44% of the patients under each treatment to develop RDS. This leads to the expected frequencies of RDS under the null hypothesis of $0.44 \times 27 = 11.93$ in the steroid group and $0.44 \times 16 = 7.07$ in the control group. The expected frequencies are presented in Table 11-2.

Note that the total expected frequencies agree with the total observed frequencies. In this case all expected frequen-

Table 11-2
Expected Frequencies of RDS

	RDS	No RDS	Total
Steroid group	11.93 (44%)	15.07	27
Control group	7.07 (44%)	8.93	16
Total	19 (44%)	24	43

cies are greater than five, and so sample size is sufficient for the chi-square test to be reliable. The chi-square statistic compares the observed frequencies with the expected frequencies, if the null were true, through the formula

$$\chi^2 = \Sigma \frac{(O) - E)^2}{E}$$

where Σ is a summation sign indicating the statistic is calculated by summing over each pair of frequencies, O represents an observed frequency, and E the corresponding expected frequency. The chi-square statistic will always be greater than or equal to zero. If the data agree with the null hypothesis, the observed and expected frequencies will be similar, the differences $(O - E)$ will be small, and the chi-square statistic will be relatively close to zero. However, if the sample disagrees with the null, then the observed frequencies will be far from the expected, and the statistic will be relatively large. For the data from the Vermont study:

$$\chi^2 = \frac{(6 - 11.93)^2}{11.93} + \frac{(21 - 15.07)^2}{15.07} + \frac{(13 - 7.07)^2}{7.07} + \frac{(3 - 8.93)^2}{8.93} = 14.19$$

How large must a chi-square statistic be for the disagreement between observed and expected to be more than can be explained by chance? In general this depends on the number of categories for the outcome being examined and the number of groups being compared, and it is measured by the "degrees of freedom" of the test. Degrees of freedom can be calculated as $(r - 1) \times (c - 1)$ where r is the number of outcome categories and c is the number of groups being compared. For the comparison of two groups on a dichotomous outcome, there is one degree of freedom and the critical values for $P < 0.05$, $P < 0.01$, $P < 0.001$ are 3.84, 6.63, and 10.82, respectively. That is, if the value of the chi-square statistic is less than 3.84, the null hypothesis is accepted. If the value of the chi-square statistic is greater than 3.84, the treatment groups differ at $P < 0.05$. If the value is greater than 6.63, the treatment groups differ at $P < 0.01$.

The data from the Vermont study show significant disagreement with the null hypothesis at $P < 0.001$ ($\chi^2 = 14.19$ is greater than 10.82), and so we conclude there is a significant difference between treatment groups. This result offers strong evidence of a difference in the incidence of RDS for the two groups and has taken sample size into account.

In contrast, the observed and expected frequencies from the California study are:

	RDS	No RDS	Total
Observed frequencies			
Steroid group	14 (17%)	66	80
Control group	17 (21%)	62	79
Total	31 (19%)	128	159
Expected frequencies			
Steroid group	15.60 (19%)	64.40	80
Control group	15.40 (19%)	63.60	79
Total	31	128	159

Here the observed and expected frequencies agree quite well, and the corresponding value of the chi-square statistic is $X^2 = 0.41$. This value is less than 3.84, and so we conclude that there is no significant difference in the rates of RDS between the two groups, $P > 0.05$. This is a weak result and does not by itself offer strong support for the hypothesis of no difference. More information needs to be presented.

Supporting the Null Hypothesis

We have seen that accepting the null hypothesis is a weak result. While the data underlying this conclusion may offer strong support for the null, it may be that the data are simply inconclusive. Additional description, incorporating sample-size considerations, is needed to evaluate the strength of the data. Both power analysis and confidence interval estimates address this issue. This section presents the basic concepts of power and confidence intervals, with emphasis on how to interpret results that might be encountered in the literature. The calculation of confidence intervals or power is discussed in most texts on medical statistics.

The purpose of a confidence interval is to give a range of likely values for some percentage, mean, or other "parameter" of a population, based on a sample result. For example, in the Melbourne study, the sample incidence of RDS for the steroid group was 57% (12 of 21). The incidence of RDS for the population of all patients given steroid treatment is expected to be close to this percentage, but this estimate is based on a sample of only 21 subjects and so may be high or low due to sampling variation. A confidence interval provides an objective description of the uncertainty in an estimate. The 0.95 confidence interval for this percentage is (36%, 78%). We are 95% certain that the underlying risk of RDS for the population receiving steroids is between 36% and 78%.

The range of the confidence interval reflects the uncertainty due to sampling. Had the sample been larger, the interval would be narrower, reflecting greater confidence in the estimate. For example, in the California study with 80 subjects in the steroid group, the incidence of RDS was 17% and the 0.95 confidence interval is (9%, 25%). The narrower interval in this case in part reflects the larger size of the sample.

The choice of 0.95 as a level of confidence was arbitrary, although conventionally the 0.90, 0.95 or 0.99 confidence levels are used. The higher the level of confidence, the wider the interval will be. For example, the 0.99 confidence interval for the Melbourne data is (30%, 86%). We can be 95% confident that the incidence of RDS is between 36% and 78%, and 99% confident that the incidence of RDS is between 30% and 86%.

Confidence intervals are perhaps most natural when estimating one parameter. However, confidence intervals can also be calculated for differences in parameters. In the Melbourne study, the difference between rates of RDS in the two treatment groups (steroid group − control group) was 58% − 57% = 1%. The 0.95 confidence interval for this difference is −26% to 28%. The 0.95 interval suggests that steroids may reduce the risk of RDS by as much as 28%, or actually increase the rate by as much as 26%. The interval is relatively wide, suggesting that the sample is too small to give a precise comparison of treatments. This study offers only weak evidence of no difference between treatments.

Similarly, the California study gives an estimated treatment difference of 21% − 17% = 4%, with a corresponding 0.95 confidence interval of (−8%, 12%). This interval is narrower than that from the Melbourne study, reflecting the larger samples. We are 95% confident that, at best, steroid treatment reduces the incidence of RDS by 12%. Some readers may still consider this statement too weak to be confident that steroid treatment does not lead to a meaningful reduction in RDS.

Power analysis is another approach to describing the strength of a nonsignificant result. Statistically, power is defined as the probability a study will lead to rejecting the null hypothesis if, in fact, the null hypothesis is false. A power argument usually assumes some difference in the populations under study and gives the probability of selecting samples that lead the investigator to conclude that the null hypothesis is false.

The interpretation of a power statement is perhaps best explained through example. The following statement pertains to the Melbourne study, with a sample of 21 steroid and 36 control patients. Suppose the incidence of RDS in the control population is 60% (this assumption is about the unknown population incidence rate, not the observed sample incidence). Suppose steroid treatment actually reduces the incidence of RDS by half, to 30%, (in the population of patients given steroids). Then a study of this size has only a 62% chance of statistically detecting the effectiveness of treatment. That is, even if steroid treatment is dramatically effective, a study of this size is too small to guarantee a high probability of showing a significant difference between treatments. The interpretation is that the sample size is too small to have much confidence in a conclusion of no difference.

If a study has reasonable power (conventionally 80%) of detecting a reasonable difference, then a conclusion of no difference can be trusted. For example, suppose a study was based on samples of 150 under each treatment and that the underlying incidence of RDS in the control population is 60%. Such a study would have an 80% chance (power of 0.80) of detecting a difference between treatments if steroids reduce the rate of RDS to 44% or less. The interpretation is that if no significant difference is observed, we are confident that steroid treatment does not reduce the incidence of RDS to less than 44%. (Some readers may consider a sample of this size too small as well.)

When emphasis is being placed on a nonsignificant result, it is the duty of the authors to give some description of the strength of the result. Both power analysis and confidence intervals can be used to address this issue. The choice of which approach to use in a particular situation is often just a matter of personal opinion. However, there is one important difference underlying the two approaches. Power analysis is based solely on the sample size of a study and does not depend on the actual sample findings. Confidence intervals are based on the observed sample data as well as sample size. Therefore, confidence intervals are often preferred when focusing on a few results, since this approach makes more complete use of the sample findings. Since it does not depend on the actual sample outcome, power may be calculated when planning a study to ensure the sample size will be adequate to trust a nonsignificant result. Also when presenting many results, a general description through power may be less confusing than presenting a great many confidence intervals.

SUMMARY

Statistical studies must be thought of as presenting evidence for, rather than proof of, some hypothesis. Studies should be read critically in order to weigh the strength of this evidence. The medical science, study design, and finally the statistical strength of the study must all be considered. Patients should be enlisted in a manner to minimize any possible bias in patient selection or assignment to treatment, and an author should address possible bias when presenting a study. Statistically, a significant result is strong evidence, while a nonsignificant result is weak evidence. If an article focuses on a nonsignificant result, the author should describe the strength of that result either through power analysis or interval estimation. Consistent findings across studies offer the strongest support for any hypothesis.

REFERENCES

1. Mead PB, Clapp JF: The use of betamethasone and timed delivery in management of premature rupture of the membranes in the preterm pregnancy. *J Reprod Med* 1977;19:3.
2. Eggers TR, Doule LW, Pepperell RJ: Premature rupture of the membranes. *Med J Aust* 1979;1:209.
3. Garite TJ, Freeman RK, Linzey EM, et al: Prospective randomized study of corticosteroids in the management of premature rupture of the membranes and premature gestation. *Am J Obstet Gynecol* 1981;141:508.

Eastern College of Nursing Library

INDEX

Abortion, induced
  maternal mortality and, 4, 12, 13
  reproductive mortality and, 55
  trends over time in, 12, 13
Abortion reporting, 10–11, 12, 13, 16
Abortion, spontaneous
  low birth weight and, 78–79
  preterm birth and, 79
  working environment and, 210, 229
Abruptio placentae, 147
Acetylcholinesterase (ACHE), 177–178
Adrenal hyperplasia, congenital, 176
Age
  gestational, *see* Gestational age
  gynecologic, and low birth weight, 73
  maternal, *see* Maternal age
  paternal, and perinatal mortality, 157
Alcoholism and alcohol use, 191, 219
Alkaline phosphatase, 178
Alpha-fetoprotein (AFP)
  amniocentesis with, 176–177
  maternal serum, 179, 182–188
Alphamethyldopa, 148
Altitude, and low birth weight, 74
American College of Obstetricians and Gynecologists (ACOG), 5, 6, 28
Amniocentesis, 174–180
  amniotic fluid tests in, 176–178
  family history and, 180
  fluid cell tests in, 175–176
  indications for, 178, 179
  limitations of, 178–179
Amniotic fluid embolism, 17
Amniotic fluid infection syndrome
  low birth weight and, 75–76
  sexual intercourse during pregnancy and, 79
Anoxia
  perinatal mortality and, 23, 24
  maternal smoking and, 78
Antihypertensive medication, 147, 148–150
Asphyxia
  effects of, 94–97
  fetal heart monitoring in, 100, 111
  gestational age and, 96
  mental retardation and, 96–97
  neurological problems and, 95–96
  perinatal mortality and, 23, 24
Asthma, 74
Auscultation, fetal, 97–98

Bacteriuria, and low birth weight, 76–77
Beta$_2$ agonists, 86
Biopsy
  chorionic villus, 173
  liver, fetal, 180
  skin, fetal, 180
Birth defects
  definition of, 211
  length of follow-up in, 211–212
  working environment and, 211–212
Birth interval, and low birth weight, 73, 74
Birth order
  low birth weight and, 73
  older gravida and, 161–162
  perinatal mortality and, 157
Birth weight
  cesarean section and, 125–126, 140
  gestational age and, 66–69
  low, *see* Low birth weight
Blacks
  cesarean section and, 129, 140
  low birth weight and, 71–73, 88
  maternal mortality and, 13–14
  older gravida and, 157–158, 160
  perinatal mortality and, 20, 23
Blood tests
  fetal, 180
  maternal, 182–188
Blue Cross, 133
Brain damage
  fetal asphyxia and, 94
  fetal heart monitoring and, 102
Breast-feeding, 233
Breech presentation
  cesarean section and, 53, 134, 135, 137–138
  short gestation and, 82

Calcium channel blockers, 86
Centers for Disease Control (CDC), 227
  birth defects and, 211, 220
  cesarean section and, 52–53
  maternal mortality and, 7, 10, 11, 14, 16, 40, 48
  perinatal mortality and, 21, 28
  reproductive mortality and, 55
Cerebral palsy, 93
  fetal asphyxia and, 95, 96–97
  fetal heart monitoring and, 101–102
Cervical incompetence, and low birth weight, 75
Cesarean section, 119–142
  benefits of, 119–120
  complications in, 134–138
  costs of, 120
  experience and trends in, 121–124
  health system factors in, 129–134
  hospital ownership and, 132
  hospital size and, 130–131
  hospital teaching status and, 130
  infant birth weight and, 125–126
  insurance coverage and, 132–134
  issues of appropriate use of, 121
  marital status and, 127
  Massachusetts study of, 49–52, 139–142

maternal age and, 125
maternal education and, 128–129
maternal residence and, 127–128
neonatal intensive care and, 131
obstetric specialization and, 131–132
population at risk for, 124–129
prenatal care and, 126–127
race and ethnicity and, 129
repeat use of, 123–124, 134, 135, 137, 138
risks and benefits of, 52–54
vaginal delivery versus, 49–52
Childbearing
causes of death in, 17
maternal mortality and, 4, 11–12, 12–13, 16, 17
regional factors in, 16
reporting in, 11–12
trends over time in, 12–13
Cholera, 247–248
Cholestasis, maternal intra-hepatic, 159
Chorioamnionitis, 75, 84
Chorionic villus biopsy, 173
Chromosomal abnormality, 212
congenital malformations and, 170
frequency of, 170
maternal serum alpha-fetoprotein (MSAFP) for, 186–187
Chromosome analysis, 175, 179
Cigarette smoking, *see* Smoking
Circulatory system disorders, maternal, 74
Class, *see* Socioeconomic status
Cleft lip and cleft palate, 171–172
Coitus, *see* Sexual intercourse
Commission on Professional and Hospital Activities (CPHA), 10, 134–135
Congenital malformations, 167–204
amniocentesis in, 174–180
chorionic villus biopsy in, 173
definition of, 168
diabetes mellitus and, 151, 155–156
epidemiology of, 170–172
etiologic classification of, 168–170
fetoscopy and fetal tissue sampling in, 180–181
maternal blood sampling in, 182–188
older gravida and, 161–162
perinatal mortality and, 23
prenatal detection of, 172–173
prevalance rates for, 171, 202–204
prevention of, 188–191
short gestation and, 82
ultrasound examination in, 181–182
Congenital rubella syndrome (CRS), 190
Contraceptives
Massachusetts study of, 59–60
reproductive mortality and, 54–55, 56, 58
Costs
cesarean section, 120
fetal heart monitoring, 113
Council of the International Federation of Obstetricians and Gynecologists (CIFOG), 145

Counseling, prepregnancy, 163
Cyanotic heart disease, 74
Cystic fibrosis, 178

Diabetes mellitus, 150–156
  degree of metabolic control
    and outcome of, 154
  low birth weight and, 74
  perinatal mortality and, 161
  prevention of, 190–191
  screening for, 163–164
Doppler ultrasound, 98
Down's syndrome, 161–162
Dystocia, and cesarean section,
    134, 135, 137, 138

Ectopic pregnancy
  maternal mortality and, 4,
    11, 12, 13, 16
  reporting, 11
  reproductive mortality and, 55
  trends over time in, 12, 13
Education, maternal, and
    cesarean section, 128–129,
    140, 141
Elderly gravida, *see* Older
    gravida
Electronic monitoring, *see*
    Fetal heart rate monitoring
Embolism, and maternal
  mortality, 16, 17
Environmental factors
  congenital malformations
    and, 170
  see also Working environment
Ethanol, and prematurity, 86
Ethnicity
  cesarean section and, 129,
    140, 141
  see also Racial factors

Family history, in amnio-
    centesis, 180
Fat, and growth in girls, 265
Fetal alcohol syndrome (FAS),
    191
Fetal death, 18
  fetal asphyxia and, 94
  see also Perinatal mortality
Fetal distress, and cesarean
    section, 134, 135, 137, 138
Fetal heart rate monitoring,
    97–111
  antepartum testing and, 111
  asphyxia effects and, 94–97
  cesarean section and, 123,
    138
  classic patterns in, 99
  clinical trials of, 100–101
  cost of, 113
  goal of, 93
  history of, 97
  needless interventions in,
    112–113
  patterns associated with
    adverse outcomes in, 102–
    103, 104–107
  perinatal mortality and, 24,
    109–110
  predictive value of, 100
  problems with, 101–102
  responses in, 103, 108, 109,
    110
  risks of, 112–113
  techniques for, 98
Fetal tissue sampling, 180–181
Fetoscopy, 180–181
Folic acid supplementation,
    189

Genetic factors
  congenital malformations
    and, 170
  low birth weight and, 71–73
  prevalence rate for, 202–204
Genetic linkage, 175–176

Genital growth in girls, 263–264
Georgia Neonatal Surveillance System, 53–54
Gestational age
  birth weight and, 66–69
  establishing length of, 65–66
  fetal asphyxia and, 96
  short, *see* Premature birth
  ultrasound examination for, 181
Girls, growth in, *see* Growth in girls
Glomerulonephritis, 75
Gravida, older, *see* Older gravida
Growth in girls, 255–269
  adipose growth in, 265
  assessment of, 259–260
  characteristic patterns in, 260–262
  first cycle of, 257–259
  genital growth in, 263–264
  in height and weight, 256
  lymphoid growth in, 264
  neural growth in, 262–263
  neuromuscular development and, 266–267
  secondary sex characteristics and, 267–269
  second cycle of, 259–260
  segmental growth in, 265
  skeletal development in, 267
Gynecologic age, and low birth weight, 73

Health care system, and cesarean section, 129–134
Health insurance plans, and cesarean section, 123, 132–134
Health maintenance organizations (HMOs), 133
Heart rate monitoring, *see* Fetal heart rate monitoring
Hemorrhage
  fetal heart monitoring and, 112
  maternal mortality and, 44
  short gestation and, 82
Hispanics
  cesarean section and, 140
  low birth weight and, 73
Hospital characteristics, and cesarean section, 130–131, 132, 141–142
Hydralazine, 148
Hydrochlorothiazide, 148
Hyperglycemia, maternal, 156, 164
Hypertension
  evaluation of, 164
  low birth weight and, 74
  medication for, 148–149
  older gravida and, 146–150
  perinatal mortality and, 158–159, 161
  premature termination of pregnancy in, 150
Hyperthyroidism, 75

Illegitimacy
  low birth weight and, 80
  short gestation and, 82
Illness of mother, and low birth weight, 74–75
Immunoglobulin (IgM), in viral infections, 77
Infant Formula Action Coalition (INFACT), 238–239
Infant formula controversies, 233–251
  coalitions against use of, 238–239
  events leading to code on, 239–243

infectious diseases and, 243–249
medical community and, 237–238
U.S. response to, 235–237, 249–250
Infarcts, placental, 147
Infections
growth cycles in girls and, 257
infant formula use and, 243–249
low birth weight and, 75–77
maternal mortality and, 44
perinatal mortality and, 24
Infecundability, and working environment, 208–209
Insurance plans, and cesarean section, 123, 132–134
Intensive care unit, neonatal, 131
Intercourse, *see* Sexual intercourse
International Code of Marketing of Breast-Milk Substitutes, 234–235; *see also* Infant formula controversies
Intrauterine growth retardation (IUGR), 66, 148

Kaiser prepaid health plan, 134

Liver biopsy, fetal, 180
Low birth weight
birth interval and, 73, 74
birth order and, 73
causes of, 69–81
cervical incompetence and, 75
cesarean section mortality in, 53, 54
cigarette smoking and, 77–78
decrease in proportion of, 87–88
genetic factors and, 71–73
illegitimacy and, 80
infant formula and, 244
maternal age and, 73
maternal illness and, 74–75
maternal infections and, 75–77
maternal nutrition and, 70–71
maternal size and, 70
multiple factor interaction in, 80
multiple gestation and, 70
neonatal and infant deaths and, 65
perinatal mortality and, 22, 69
prevention of, 86–87
previous spontaneous loss and, 79
sexual intercourse during pregnancy and, 79–80
short gestation and, 82
Lupus erythematosis, 74
Lymphoid growth in girls, 264

Malpractice, 123
Marital status, and cesarean section, 127
Massachusetts Medical Society Committee on Maternal Welfare study
causes of death in, 43–45
cesarean section mortality in, 49–52
creation of, 36
National Center for Health Statistics (NCHS) data versus, 39–43
oral contraceptives in, 59–60

physician interview in, 37–38
reproductive mortality in, 58–60
results of, 39–54
use of data from, 47–49
Maternal age
cesarean section and, 125
low birth weight and, 73
perinatal mortality rate and, 22–23
short gestation and, 81, 82
see also Older gravida
Maternal death
definition of, 4–5, 61
direct and indirect, 5
Maternal illness, and low birth weight, 74–75
Maternal intrahepatic cholestasis, 159
Maternal mortality, 3–17, 25, 35–62
abortion reporting and, 10–11
causes of death in, 16–17, 43–45
childbearing mortality reporting in, 11–12
conditions associated with, 40
data sources for, 7–12
declines in, 1, 2
definitions of, 1, 3–6, 61
diabetes mellitus and, 151
ectopic pregnancy reporting and, 11
epidemiology of, 12–17
historical perspective on, 36
Massachusetts study of, 37–39
maternal characteristics in, 13–16
preventability of, 45–47
racial differences in, 13–14
regional factors in, 14–16
surveillance in, 10–12
trends over time in, 12–13
uses of rates in, 6
vital records on, 7–10
see also Reproductive mortality
Maternal serum alpha-fetoprotein (MSAFP), 183–188
cost-effectiveness of, 185–186
high, 183–186
low, 186–188
Maternal stress, and prematurity, 81
Maternal weight
low birth weight and, 70–71
short gestation and, 81
Medicaid, and cesarean section, 133
Menarche, 268–269
Mental retardation, 93, 212
asphyxia and, 96–97
fetal heart monitoring and, 101–102
Metabolic disorders, 175
Methyldopa, 148
Midforceps delivery, 123
Miscarriage, and working environment, 210
Monitoring, fetal heart, *see* Fetal heart rate monitoring
Mortality rates, *see* Maternal mortality; Perinatal mortality; Reproductive mortality
Mother, *see* Maternal *headings*
Multigravida, *see* Older gravida
Multivitamin supplementation, 189

National Center for Health Statistics (NCHS)

Massachusetts study versus, 39–43
maternal mortality and, 5, 7, 10, 11, 12, 54
perinatal mortality and, 21, 23
working environment and, 208, 209
National Hospital Discharge Survey, 11
National Infant Mortality Survey, 21, 25
National Institute for Occupational Safety and Health, 227
National Institutes of Health, 121
Neonatal deaths, 18
cigarette smoking and, 78
fetal asphyxia and, 94
recent reductions in, 87–88
see also Perinatal mortality
Neonatal intensive care unit, 131
Neural growth in girls, 262–263
Neural tube defects (NTDs), 212
amniocentesis for, 174, 176–177, 180
maternal serum alpha-fetoprotein (MSAFP) and, 183, 184–185
population differences in, 172
prevention of, 189
Neurological problems, and fetal asphyxia, 95, 96
Neuromuscular growth in girls, 266–267
Nicotine, 78
Nonpreventable death, definition for, 62
Nutrition, maternal
low birth weight and, 70–71
prematurity prevention and, 86

Occupational factors, *see* Working environment
Older gravida, 145–164
age definition in, 145
diabetes mellitus in, 150–156
hypertension and, 146–150
perinatal mortality and, 156–162
socioeconomic status and, 157–158
Oral contraceptives, *see* Contraceptives
Oxygen, fetal, and maternal smoking, 78

Patent ductus arteriosus, 220
Paternal age, and perinatal mortality, 157
Perinatal mortality, 18–24, 25–28
amniotic fluid infection syndrome and, 75–76
causes of death in, 23–24
data sources for, 20–21
definitions for, 18–20
diabetes mellitus and, 151, 154, 156–157
epidemiology of, 21–24
fetal heart monitoring and, 109–111
hypertension and, 147–148, 150
low birth weight and, 69
maternal factors in, 22–23
older gravida and, 156–162
overlap between neonatal deaths and, 21–22
trends over time in, 21–22

Placental growth retardation, 147
Preeclampsia, and hypertension, 148, 158–159, 161
Premature rupture of membrane
  epidemiology of, 84
  statistical study of, 274–278, 284–287
Prematurity
  causes of, 81–82
  clinical contexts of, 82–84
  diabetes mellitus and, 156
  fetal asphyxia and, 94
  iatrogenic, 78
  induced abortion and, 78–79
  maternal stress and, 81
  prevention of, 86–87
  see also Preterm birth
Prenatal care
  cesarean section and, 126–127, 140
  low birth weight and, 78
  prematurity and, 86
  public awareness of need for, 164
Preterm birth
  classification of, 68–69
  defining problem in, 65–69
  epidemiology of, 65–88
  gestational age and birth weight in, 66–69
  gestational length determination in, 65–66
  see also Prematurity
Preventable death, definition of, 62
Primigravida, *see* Older gravida

Racial factors
  cesarean section and, 129, 140, 141
  low birth weight and, 71–73
  maternal mortality and, 13–14, 16
Renal disease, maternal, 74
Reproductive mortality, 54–60
  Massachusetts study of, 58–60
  oral contraceptives and, 54–55
Residence, and cesarean section, 127–128
Respiratory distress syndrome
  diabetes mellitus and, 151, 156
  older gravida and, 160
  perinatal mortality and, 23, 24
Rubella vaccination, 189–190

Screening programs
  congenital malformations in, 172–173
  diabetes mellitus and, 163–164
  hypertension and, 164
  maternal blood sampling in, 182–188
  see also Amniocentesis
Secondary sex characteristics in girls, 267–269
Sexual intercourse
  low birth weight and, 79–80
  premature rupture of membranes and, 84
Skeletal growth in girls, 267
Skin biopsy, fetal, 180
Smoking
  low birth weight and, 77–78, 86
  oral contraceptives and, 60
  short gestation and, 81
  toxic agents in work environment and, 219

Socioeconomic status
  cesarean section and, 128–129, 141
  low birth weight and, 88
  older gravida and, 157–158, 160
  perinatal mortality and, 23
  short gestation and, 81
Sperm evaluation, 212–213
Spontaneous abortion, *see* Abortion, spontaneous
Statistics, 273–298
  analysis in, 287–289
  chi-square test of independence in, 290–294
  evaluation of, 278–298
  null hypothesis in, 295–298
  premature rupture of membrane (PROM) example in, 274–278
  study design in, 280–283
Sterilization, 55, 56
Stress, and prematurity, 81

Tocolytic therapy, and prematurity, 86–87
Toxemia, 44, 148
Toxic agents in working environment, 213–219
  list of agents in, 214–218
  research on, 219–220
Trisomy, 21, 186, 187

Ultrasound examination, 181–182
UNICEF, 240
Urinary infections, maternal, 75

Video display terminals (VDTs), 221–227
Viral infections, and low birth weight, 77
Vital statistics, 25
  maternal mortality and, 7–10
  perinatal mortality and, 20–21
  underreporting in, 7

Weight
  birth, *see* Birth weight; Low birth weight
  growth in girls', 256
  maternal, *see* Maternal weight
Whites
  cesarean section and, 129
  low birth weight and, 71–73
  maternal mortality and, 13–14
Working environment, 205–230
  assessing reproductive impairment in, 208–213
  birth defects and, 210–212
  exposure and outcome indices in, 229
  future studies in, 227–229
  infecundability and, 208–209
  occupational history and, 206–208
  pregnancy loss and, 210–211
  reproduction and, 205–206
  research on, 219–221
  surveillance of, 220–221
  toxic agents in, 213–219
  video display terminals (VDTs) example in, 221–227
World Health Organization (WHO)
  infant formula controversies and, 233–251
  maternal mortality and, 5, 18, 20

LIBRARY
WESTERN COLLEGE
OF NURSING & MIDWIFERY
GARTNAVEL COMPLEX
1053 GREAT WESTERN ROAD
GLASGOW G12